Shared Care Glaucoma

A Clinical Text for Ophthalmic Allied Professionals

Amar Alwitry

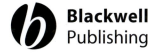

Blackwell
Publishing

This edition first published 2000
© 2008 by Amar Alwitry

Blackwell Publishing was acquired by John Wiley & Sons in February 2007. Blackwell's publishing programme has been merged with Wiley's global Scientific, Technical, and Medical business to form Wiley-Blackwell.

Registered office
John Wiley & Sons Ltd, The Atrium, Southern Gate, Chichester, West Sussex, PO19 8SQ, United Kingdom

Editorial office
9600 Garsington Road, Oxford, OX4 2DQ, United Kingdom

For details of our global editorial offices, for customer services and for information about how to apply for permission to reuse the copyright material in this book please see our website at www.wiley.com/ wiley-blackwell.

Library of Congress Cataloging-in-Publication Data

Alwitry, Amar.
Shared care glaucoma : a clinical text for ophthalmic allied professionals / Amar Alwitry.
p. ; cm.
Includes bibliographical references and index.
ISBN-13: 978-1-4051-6800-7 (pbk. : alk. paper)
ISBN-10: 1-4051-6800-5 (pbk. : alk. paper) 1. Glaucoma. 2. Ophthalmic assistants. 3. Health care teams. I. Title.
[DNLM: 1. Glaucoma. 2. Ophthalmology. 3. Optometry. 4. Orthoptics. 5. Patient Care Team. 6. Specialties, Nursing.
WW 290 A4775s 2008]
RE871.A48 2008
617.7′41–dc22
2007040600

A catalogue record for this book is available from the British Library.

Set in 10/12 pt Sabon by SNP Best-set Typesetter Ltd., Hong Kong
Printed in Singapore by Fabulous Printers Pte Ltd

1 2008

Contents

Foreword

Modern glaucoma management could be defined as a mixture of art and science. Under the 'art' umbrella reside skills in communication, predicting the future, bespoke care and conveying a positive attitude (glaucoma diagnosis alone is linked with reduced self-assessed quality of life). Within 'science' we have individual and cohort data analysis, risk assessment, general and ocular physiology, pathology and evidence-based intervention strategy determination.

The days of 'repeat drops, see two months' should be long gone as those ophthalmologists with a glaucoma interest strive to practise holistic medicine to maximize their patients' quality of life. Good glaucoma care takes time to learn and to deliver, a sound-bite well known to glaucomatologists, but its wisdom is often lost on non-clinicians.

In order to satisfy the constant pressures within the service, now so often target driven, glaucoma care is being 'shared' with non-ophthalmologists. This book is aimed at that constantly growing band of 'ocular health professionals' (optometrists, ophthalmic nurses and orthoptists) who are called upon to extend their traditional role into the realm of what, in the past, was the doctors'. This can be safely and successfully achieved by additional training which, in my opinion, is best executed in an apprenticed-based scenario within a specialist-led glaucoma clinic. Mr. Alwitry rightly states that glaucoma care should be under the overall control of an ophthalmologist. His book encourages high-quality shared care and not autonomous non-physician led care.

The essence of good medicine is making good decisions. To do this well in a chronic degenerative condition that is predominantly treated medically, one requires knowledge of the range of normality, the natural history patterns of the disease process, relevant pharmacology, psychology, and the interpretation of disease progression markers.

Mr Alwitry's distillation of the important features of glaucoma detection and management is well timed in this era of rapid change. It uses a relaxed narrative style with much 'common sense' to impart the necessary knowledge and skills required of the non-ophthalmologist working in a high-quality glaucoma service. It covers the majority of the syllabus for each of the College of Optometrists Glaucoma diplomas (A and B) and I am sure will become a core text for those studying for these and other examinations as well as for 'fully trained' ophthalmologists who wish to improve their understanding and practice of glaucoma management. It can be 'skim read' for a flavor of what is required, but the real value of the book is in its attention to detail. Frequently asked questions are anticipated and a logical response given, supported by evidence from the plethora of recent peer-reviewed literature, where it exists. There are, however, often no clear right and wrong decisions within many individuals' glaucoma management plans and this is well recognised and conveyed in the book.

What is offered here is a diet of well tempered gems, distilled from Amar's experience and a realistic appraisal of the literature. It now tops my list as essential reading for those new (and not so new) to my glaucoma service and its associated hospital- and community-based shared care schemes.

Stephen A Vernon
DM FRCS FRCOphth DO
Consultant Ophthalmologist
University Hospital
Nottingham

Acknowledgments

I would like to thank my previous trainers Mr Stephen Vernon and Mr Anthony King for their kind support and mentorship.

Thanks also to David Bennett and Belinda Hughes (shared care optometrists) and Julie Huntbach (fellow ophthalmologist) for taking time to read the text and give their invaluable (and brutally honest) opinion.

Chapter 1

Introduction

The population is continually growing with more people living longer. We are also detecting more glaucoma meaning that the volume of patients needing our care is escalating rapidly. In an ideal world we would expand the hospital eye service to cope with this added burden, however, in the modern socioeconomic climate it is impossible to keep up. We clearly need to look at other options. As ophthalmologists we are fortunate to have a massive workforce of eye professionals who are allied to us. Optometrists, orthoptists and ophthalmic nurse specialists are all highly skilled professionals in their own right and it makes sense to utilize their knowledge and skills to care for glaucoma patients.

It is unreasonable to expect allied professionals to venture out and try to manage glaucoma patients alone. They are not specifically trained for it and thus moving the glaucoma load on to their shoulders without the support of an ophthalmologist who is trained in glaucoma is a concern. Even with appropriate training, professionals need to have the benefit of continual professional development. They need to remain up to date and have the opportunity to ask questions and challenge themselves with harder cases.

It is my genuine feeling that all glaucoma shared care should be undertaken under the umbrella of a professional specifically trained to provide specialist glaucoma care, i.e. a consultant ophthalmologist. Not only are consultant ophthalmologists trained in glaucoma but they also understand and are able to deal with the whole spectrum of ophthalmology. Taking this key individual out of the loop will lead to significant patient safety concerns – it is not fair on the patient and it is not fair on the clinician who is left to manage them without the back-up of someone who is specifically trained to concentrate on glaucoma. We all have a duty of care to our patients to give them the best that we can. Having one's glaucoma managed by an experienced and competent consultant ophthalmologist with glaucoma as their special interest is clearly the best one can hope for. This is not a realistic proposition in this day and age. We need to expand and evolve and work as a team to deliver an excellent level of care. We can only do this by working together. The shared care professional works with the glaucoma specialist and the glaucoma specialist in turn offers adequate training in the first instance and also a commitment to ensuring standards and continuing professional development of the clinicians under their supervision.

This book cannot be used in isolation. Formal training in the management of the glaucoma patient is required before one can embark upon managing glaucoma patients. This applies to every branch of healthcare professional, be they nurse practitioner or ophthalmologist. As part of their training ophthalmologists need to undergo 6 months dedicated training in managing glaucoma patients before they are deemed competent enough to manage glaucoma as a generalist. When faced with complicated glaucoma the general ophthalmologist or ophthalmologist with another special interest freely refers to the glaucoma specialist. Without appropriate training, supervision and back-up how can a shared care professional hope to do the best by their patient?

Shared care programs should ideally be run under the umbrella and overall control of a consultant ophthalmologist with a special interest in glaucoma. Anything less risks patient safety. It is not ego or pride but simply a matter of logic – it is after all what we are trained for. I would not suggest that an ophthalmologist run an optometric practice without the help of an optometrist. We each have our specialities and by working as a team we can all pull together and manage glaucoma well. We need to enhance the primary and secondary care interface and work together utilizing appropriate protocols and maximize the quality of care we provide with our limited resources.

This text gives you the basics. Glaucoma management is an art rather than a science and as your confidence and experience grows you will come to find your own feet with regard to managing your patients. I hope this text helps.

My sole aim is to help everyone manage glaucoma to the best of their abilities.

Abbreviations used throughout

AAC: acute angle closure
AACG: acute angle-closure glaucoma
AC: anterior chamber
ACG: angle-closure glaucoma
AGIS: Advanced Glaucoma Intervention Study
ALT: argon laser trabeculoplasty
CAC: chronic angle closure
CACG: chronic angle-closure glaucoma
CB: ciliary body
CCT: central corneal thickness
CDR: cup-to-disc ratio
CRVO: central retinal vein occlusion
CSLO: confocal scanning laser ophthalmoscope
DCT: dynamic contour tonometer
DR: diabetic retinopathy
EMGT: Early Manifest Glaucoma Trial
FDT/P: frequency doubling technology/perimetry
GAT: Goldmann applanation tonometry
GCP: glaucoma change probability
GDD: glaucoma drainage device
GHT: glaucoma hemifield test
GLT: Glaucoma Laser Trial
ICE: iridocorneal endothelial syndrome
IOP: intraocular pressure
LASIK: laser in-situ keratomileusis

LPI: laser peripheral iridotomy
LTF: long-term fluctuation
MMT: maximal medical therapy
NFI: nerve fiber index
NRR: neuroretinal rim
NSAIDs: non-steroidal anti-inflammatory drugs
NTG: normal-tension glaucoma
NTGS: Normal-Tension Glaucoma Study
OAG: open-angle glaucoma
OCT: optical coherence tomography
ODH: optic disc hemorrhage
OHT: ocular hypertension
OHTS: Ocular Hypertension Treatment Study
ONH: optic nerve head
ORA: ocular response analyzer
PAC: primary angle closure
PACG: primary angle-closure glaucoma
PAS: peripheral anterior synechiae
PC: posterior chamber
PDS: pigmentary dispersion syndrome
PLR: pointwise linear regression
PXE: pseudoexfoliation
PPA: peripapillary atrophy
RBT: rebound tonometer
RNFL: retinal nerve fiber layer
RPE: retinal pigment epithelium
SITA: Swedish interactive threshold algorithm
SL: Schwalbe's line
SLP: scanning laser polarimetry
SLT: selective laser trabeculoplasty
TCA: topographic change analysis
TM: trabecular meshwork
VCC: variable corneal compensation
vCDR: vertical cup-to-disc ratio

Section 1

About Glaucoma

This section will take you through the basics about glaucoma and give you an understanding of the nature of the beast we are dealing with and how we examine and assess our glaucoma patients. This is arguably the most important section, as without an understanding of glaucoma and how it affects the individual patient we cannot hope to formulate effective management plans.

Chapter 2

Epidemiology and risk factors for glaucoma

Why should I read this chapter?

Epidemiology is not boring and this chapter will not shove endless numbers at you. It is important to understand the scope of the problem we are facing when aiming to anticipate the level of care we will have to provide for our patients. This chapter will explain the epidemiology of glaucoma and where we are heading as regards the numbers of patients we can hope to see in the future.

It would be ideal if we could predict which individual will develop glaucoma based upon a tick box list of risk factors. The current state of our understanding is not yet up to the task; however, as the volume and quality of data expands, we do have some clues as to what factors broadly increase the risk of a patient having or subsequently developing glaucoma. By understanding and being aware of these risk factors we may target specific patient groups and increase our rate of picking up disease. Moreover when assessing an individual patient our level of index of suspicion may be affected by the presence or absence of specific risk factors thereby affecting management.

Scope of the problem

Half of those individuals affected with glaucoma may not even be aware that they have it. Glaucoma is thought to be the third leading cause of blindness worldwide so it is an immensely important issue to tackle head on. Afrocaribbean patients will predominantly shoulder the burden of this initially silent disorder, both in terms of the numbers who get it, and the proportion subsequently blinded by it.

By 2010, 60 million people will have OAG and ACG, and glaucoma will be 'upgraded' to the second leading cause of world blindness.[1] In 2002 OAG was estimated to affect 2.22 million people over the age of 40 years in the United States[2]; it is predicted that this will rise to 2.79 million people by 2010.[1] Likewise, it was estimated that 9.4 million Chinese people had OAG and ACG in 2001.[3] This figure will inevitably rise dramatically.

These numbers are staggering and underpin the need for a robust glaucoma management infrastructure to handle the increasing workload anticipated in the not too distant future.

Naturally these estimates are based upon quantifying the number of people having a diagnosis of glaucoma. It must be made clear that counting those with a diagnosis of glaucoma does not mean that everyone else does not have the disease. Inevitably we will miss a significant proportion of patients who have silent disease. Definite disease is not quite as clear-cut as it sounds, as even glaucoma specialists can get it wrong and diagnostic uncertainty can persist (as this text will demonstrate).

Over 80% of those with ACG live in Asia, while OAG disproportionately affects those of Afrocaribbean ancestry. Women are more affected by glaucoma because of their greater prevalence of PAC, as well as their relatively greater longevity.

Over 8.4 million people will be bilaterally blind from primary glaucoma in 2010, rising to 11.1 million by 2020.[1] Previous estimates based on blindness prevalence surveys[4] suggested that 12% of world blindness (4.4 million people) was caused by glaucoma.

Glaucoma is a big problem, second only to cataract as a cause of visual morbidity worldwide. We can intervene to prevent this visual loss and thus it is clearly important to improve diagnosis and therapeutic approaches to optimize outcome in both the developed and developing world.

Prevalence

Many epidemiologic studies have documented the prevalence of POAG throughout various regions of the world.[5-18] Early studies tended to concentrate on raised IOP as the defining criterion for glaucoma but as our understanding of the disease has evolved we have sensibly moved forward to encompass other defining criteria such as visual field loss. Again the studies suffer from deficiencies in accurate diagnosis and pick-up rate of glaucoma.

Estimates of POAG prevalence among white populations have ranged between 1.1% and 2.1%.[5-9,12,13] It is clear that Afrocaribbeans have a much greater prevalence of POAG with an linear increase in age-linked prevalence starting to rise after 40 years of age.[6]

Population-based data on glaucoma in Asia has suggested a higher proportion of ACG, however generalizations are flawed as the Asian population is highly heterogeneous in nature. The Japanese Glaucoma Survey[9] found a prevalence of only 0.34% for ACG, a figure which is significantly lower than that found amongst Eskimos[19] or in some portions of China.[15,20]

Incidence

The Barbados Eye Study reported a 4-year risk of OAG of 2.2% in Afrocaribbean participants.[21] A glaucoma annual incidence of between 0.19% and 0.24% was previously reported in a white population in Sweden.[22]

Risk factors

Patterns of disease in glaucoma are not clear-cut and it is evident that it is multifactorial and multicausal. We know and suspect the presence of several risk factors which help us target specific patients and hopefully improve our diagnostic accuracy and our ability to detect disease early.

What we know

IOP

Purists argue that the link between IOP and glaucomatous optic neuropathy is not concrete; despite these views, however, there remains considerable scientific evidence supporting IOP as an ocular risk factor for POAG. More importantly it is the only risk factor we can actively and easily modify to change a patient's glaucoma. The majority of population-based prevalence studies have confirmed higher glaucoma prevalences with increasing IOP.

In the Baltimore Eye Survey[6], 10.3% of subjects with an IOP of 22 mmHg or higher had glaucoma versus only 1.2% of subjects with IOP of 21 mmHg or lower.[23] This represents an 8.6 times relative risk of glaucoma for patients with a higher IOP compared with the lower IOP group. A similar relative risk of 7.5 was found in the Barbados Eye Study[21] for patients with a raised IOP.

The incidence of glaucoma damage increases from approximately 3% in patients with an IOP between 21 and 25 mmHg, to more than 50% in patients whose IOP is higher than 35 mmHg.[24,25] The incidence of POAG is five times higher in patients with an IOP greater than 21 mmHg than in those patients with IOP lower than 21 mmHg.[16] Patients with an IOP higher than 25 mmHg have twice the incidence of glaucomatous damage compared with patients with an IOP lower than 25 mmHg.[27]

Interestingly, despite the above statistics, most patients with an IOP greater than 21 mmHg never progress to glaucomatous optic neuropathy. Conversely, some patients with an IOP consistently less than 22 mmHg ('normal' IOP) have glaucoma damage (normal-tension glaucoma). One half of the patients classified in the Baltimore Eye Survey as having demonstrable and reproducible visual-field loss consistent with glaucoma had an initial IOP below 21 mmHg.[6] Many of these patients did go on to have a high IOP on follow-up visits, however, approximately one fifth of these glaucoma patients never exhibited an above normal IOP.

Age

The prevalence of POAG increases with increasing age.[28] The Barbados Eye Study found POAG incidence rates increased from 1.2% at ages 40–49 years to 4.2% at ages of 70 years or more.[21] One study reported that the risk of developing POAG in persons older than 60 years was seven times greater than that in those younger than 40 years.[29] In white people between the ages of 43 and 54, the reported prevalence is 0.9%, while among those older than 75 years, the prevalence increases to 4.7%.[30]

Although PAC may occur at any age, it is most often first seen in the 50–65-year-old age group and analysis indicates that the risk of developing PAC increases with age.[31,32] ACG occurs in eyes that have a short axial length and reduced anterior chamber angle depth.[33] The increased incidence with age is probably explained by anatomical changes such as thickening of the lens with subsequent forward displacement of pupil architecture (see Chapter 22).

Race

Different racial groups appear to have varying prevalences of glaucoma with clear evidence that Afrocaribbeans have a disproportionately high rate of POAG compared with white people. The Baltimore Eye Survey found the prevalence of glaucoma in African Americans to be four to five times greater than that of white people.[23] Glaucoma occurs at a younger age in African Americans compared to white people, and, at the time of diagnosis, they have a greater cupping, a higher IOP, and a worse visual field.[23,34,35] In addition to being more likely to have glaucoma, they tend to progress faster, are more resistant to treatment and are more likely to go blind.[36] Clearly, they are a special group of glaucoma patients who require particular care and aggressive treatment. Although the studies described mainly African Americans it is reasonable to extrapolate the data to the black community living in Europe. Their circumstance highlights the need to understand risk factors and epidemiology of glaucoma to tailor clinical care to the individual.

When considering PAC, research indicates that approximately 0.2% of white people will suffer an angle-closure attack. The incidence of angle-closure attacks among black people is rare, but the incidence of CACG is equal to that in white people. The risk of developing ACG is higher than the risk of POAG in Southeast Asians, Japanese, North American Eskimos, and adults in the Philippines.[37,38]

Genetics/family history

The search for a single or set of genetic markers linked with POAG has met with some success. It is an on-going and exciting area of active research, and already it is clear that familial factors play a definite role in glaucoma.[39,40] Data from the population-based Rotterdam Study indicated a life-time risk of glaucoma of 22.4% in relatives of patients versus 2.3% in the relatives of the control group.[12]

These findings were reinforced by two other large population-based studies.[41,42] In a well designed prospective study by Vernon's group[39] siblings of known glaucoma patients were screened, finding an 11.8% prevalence of glaucoma in this asymptomatic group. When Vernon's group examined the normal siblings again a mean of 7 years later they found 7% had developed definite glaucoma while 19.1% were deemed glaucoma suspects. They calculated a lifetime risk to siblings of development of glaucoma of approximately 20% by age 70.

There is also evidence to suggest that the familial form of glaucoma may be more aggressive than the sporadic variety[43], highlighting this group for particular interest.

What we think

Refractive status

In the early 1980s the association between myopia and POAG was noted.[44,45] One large population-based study found a twofold to threefold increased prevalence of POAG among myopic compared with non-myopic subjects.[46] Another study[44] found that in a group of patients with POAG there were four times as many myopes than in a similar age-matched sample of the US population. They also found a higher incidence of OHT and NTG in patients with myopia.

The Blue Mountain Eye Study found an increased risk of glaucoma among patients with moderate to high myopia (>3 diopters), and a borderline risk for low myopia (<3 diopters).[46] One further study[47] found that persons younger than 35 years with more than 3 diopters of myopia had a higher prevalence of POAG.

There are some concerns regarding the findings of the various studies because myopes are more likely to have regular ophthalmic or optometric assessments and thus the pick-up rate of glaucoma will inevitably be higher with the propensity to skew the prevalence outcomes in this select group. Despite these reservations it is generally accepted that there is indeed a link between myopia and POAG.

It is possible that the abnormal collagen and connective tissue elements found in myopic patients may predispose to pathology at the lamina cribrosa and at the optic nerve head.

PAC occurs more frequently in hypermetropic eyes with shorter axial lengths and shallow ACs due to the inherent anatomical pathogenesis which underlies this condition.

Disc hemorrhages

Disc hemorrhages are found in the normal population, however there is a much greater prevalence in patients with glaucoma.[48] There is reasonably consistent evidence suggesting that glaucoma patients developing ODHs tend to progress more than patients who do not exhibit this finding.[49-50] The occurrence of an ODH was associated with an increased risk of developing a POAG end point in participants in the OHTS.[52]

Large cup-to-disc ratio

This risk factor remains in the 'what we think' section. We know that if you have a very large CDR with obvious loss of neuroretinal rim then the likelihood of glaucoma is high. However, a large CDR per se is not always pathological. Disc size has an important part to play in the assessment of the degree of optic disc cupping and the subsequent risk of glaucoma (see Chapter 7).

Diabetes

There is still uncertainty as to whether there is a link between diabetes and glaucoma. Several large and respected studies have found a link [52-54] whereas others have not.[11,23,55]

The Beaver Dam Eye Study[53] found glaucoma to be more prevalent among diabetics than in those without the disease (4.2% versus 2.0%). When persons with a history of glaucoma treatment were included in the analysis, the number of persons with diabetes was two times higher than in those without (7.8% versus 3.9%).

The Blue Mountain Eye Study[56] showed a 5.5% prevalence of glaucoma in those with diabetes compared with 2.8% prevalence in those without, with an age–gender-adjusted odds ratio of 2 to 1. Ocular hypertension was also more common in persons with diabetes (6.7%) than in those without (3.5%).

The Rotterdam Study[52] found a threefold increased association with high pressure OAG compared with non-diabetic persons. This difference was not present for the NTG group.

Interestingly, a recent paper looking at the data from the same study population disputes this link.[57]

It may be theorized that the microvasculopathy associated with diabetes can result in compromised vascular perfusion to the optic nerve head exacerbating or potentially facilitating the onset of glaucoma.

Again caution must be used when interpreting these studies as diabetics (like myopes) are more likely to attend for eye screening and therefore the pick-up rate of glaucoma may be higher.

What we're not so sure about

Hypertension

Just as with diabetes, there have been many conflicting reports with regard to the possible association between systemic hypertension and glaucoma.[52] One team of researchers found a link between the two[23] however this link was not clear-cut. They found that young people with systemic hypertension are less likely than non-hypertensive people of the same age group to develop glaucoma. However among the elderly, hypertension does become a significant risk factor for the development of glaucoma.[56,58] It is reasonable to assume that age-related changes in microvasculature and changes in autoregulation may have some implication for optic nerve head blood flow and glaucomatous optic neuropathy.

What is more clear is the role of nocturnal dips in blood pressure and the risk of progression of glaucoma[59] particularly in normal-tension glaucoma patients with apparently pressure-independent disease (see Chapter 20).

Hypothyroidism

Two studies[60,61] reported a statistically significant association between hypothyroidism and POAG. It is thought that hypothyroidism causes accumulation of hyaluronic acid in the trabecular meshwork increasing IOP by decreasing aqueous outflow.

Vasospastic disorders

It has been suggested that individuals who suffer from migraine or Raynaud's phenomenon (exposure to cold or strong emotion triggering vascular spasm resulting in interruption of blood flow to the fingers, toes, ears or nose) may be at an increased risk of developing glaucoma, particularly NTG. The vasoconstriction associated with these disorders could potentially lead to decreased perfusion of the optic nerve head and an increased risk of glaucoma.

Phelps and Corbett documented an increased frequency of both migraine in patients with NTG as compared with normals, OHT and patients with high-pressure glaucoma.[62] The Blue Mountain Eye Study suggested a possible association between typical migraine and OAG.[63] Both the Beaver Dam Eye Study[64] and another study[65] failed to confirm this association. The Collaborative Normal-Tension Glaucoma Study[66] indicated that NTG patients with migraine may progress at a greater rate than those without migraine, potentially indicating a worse prognosis.

One recent study[67] assessed the prevalence of migraine finding that it was indeed significantly more common in patients with NTG compared to control patients and patients with high-pressure glaucoma.

References

1. Quigley HA, Broman AT. The number of people with glaucoma worldwide in 2010 and 2020. Br J Ophthalmol 2006; 90: 262–267.
2. Friedman DS, Wolfs RC, O'Colmain BJ, Klein BE, Taylor HR, West S, Leske MC, Mitchell P, Congdon N, Kempen J. Eye Diseases Prevalence Research Group. Prevalence of open-angle glaucoma among adults in the United States. Arch Ophthalmol 2004; 122: 532–538.
3. Foster PJ, Johnson GJ. Glaucoma in China: how big is the problem? Br J Ophthalmol 2001; 85: 1277–1282.
4. Resnikoff S, Pascolini D, Etya'ale D, *et al.* Global data on visual impairment in the year 2002. Bull World Health Organ 2004; 82: 844–851.
5. Ekstrom C. Prevalence of open-angle glaucoma in Central Sweden: The Tierp Glaucoma Survey. Acta Ophthalmol Scand 1996; 74: 107–112.
6. Tielsch JM, Sommer A, Katz J, *et al.* Racial variations in the prevalence of primary open-angle glaucoma: The Baltimore Eye Survey. JAMA 1991; 266: 369–374.
7. Klein BEK, Klein R, Sponsel W, *et al.* Prevalence of glaucoma: The Beaver Dam Eye Study. Ophthalmology 1992; 99: 1499–1504.
8. Coffey M, Reidy A, Wormaid R, *et al.* Prevalence of glaucoma in the West of Ireland. Br J Ophthalmol 1993; 77: 17–21.
9. Shiose Y, Kitazawa Y, Tsukahara S, *et al.* Epidemiology of glaucoma in Japan: A nationwide glaucoma survey. Jpn J Ophthalmol 1991; 35: 133–155.
10. Mason RP, Kosoko O, Wilson MR, *et al.* National survey of the prevalence and risk factors of glaucoma in St. Lucia West Indies: I. Prevalence findings. Ophthalmology 1989; 65: 1363–1368.
11. Leske MC, Connell A, Schachat A, *et al.* The Barbados Eye Study: Prevalence of open-angle glaucoma. Arch Ophthalmol 1994; 112: 821–829.
12. Dielemars I, Vingerling J, Wolfs R, *et al.* The prevalence of primary open-angle glaucoma in a population-based study in the Netherlands: The Rotterdam Study. Ophthalmology 1994; 101: 1851–1855.
13. Mitchell P, Smith W, Attebo K, Healey P. Prevalence of open-angle glaucoma in Australia. Ophthalmology 1996; 103: 1661–1669.
14. Bonomi L, Marchini G, Marraffa M, *et al.* Prevalence of glaucoma and intraocular pressure distribution in a defined population: The Egna-Neumarkt Study. Ophthalmology 1998; 105: 209–215.
15. Foster P, Oen F, Machin D, *et al.* The prevalence of glaucoma in Chinese residents of Singapore: A cross-sectional population survey of the Tanjong Pagar District. Arch Ophthalmol 2000; 118: 1105–1111.
16. Foster P, Baasanhu J, Alsbirk P, *et al.* Glaucoma in Mongolia: A population-based survey in Hovsgol Province, Northern Mongolia. Arch Ophthalmol 1996; 114: 1235–1241.
17. Salmon J, Mermoud A, Ivey A, *et al.* The prevalence of primary angle closure glaucoma and open angle glaucoma in Mamre, Western Cape, South Africa. Arch Ophthalmol 1993; 111: 1263–1269.
18. Dandona L, Dandona R, Srinivas M, *et al.* Open-angle glaucoma in an urban population in Southern India: The Andhra Pradesh Eye Disease Study. Ophthalmology 2000; 107: 1702–1709.

19. Arkell SM, Lightman DA, Sommer A, *et al*. The prevalence of glaucoma among Eskimos of Northwest Alaska. Arch Ophthalmol 1987; 105: 482–485.
20. Hu Z, Zhao Z, Dong FT, *et al*. An epidemiologic investigation of glaucoma in Beijing City and Shun-yi County. Chin J Ophthalmol 1989; 25: 115.
21. Leske M, Connell A, Wu S, *et al*. Incidence of open-angle glaucoma: The Barbados Eye Studies. Arch Ophthalmol 2001; 119: 89–95.
22. Bengtsson B. Incidence of manifest glaucoma. Br J Ophthalmol 1989; 73: 483–487.
23. Tielsch J, Katz J, Quigley H, *et al*. Diabetes, intraocular pressure, and primary open-angle glaucoma in the Baltimore Eye Survey. Ophthalmology 1995; 102: 48–53.
24. Pohjanpelto PEJ, Palva J. Ocular hypertension and glaucomatous optic nerve damage. Acta Ophthalmol 1974; 52: 194.
25. Kass MA, Hart WM Jr, Gordon M, Miller JP. Risk factors favoring the development of glaucomatous visual field loss in ocular hypertension. Surv Ophthalmol 1980; 25: 155.
26. Armaly MF, Krueger D, Maundes L, *et al*. Bio-statistical analysis of the Collaborative Glaucoma Study. I. Summary report of the risk factors for glaucomatous visual-field defects. Arch Opthamol 1980; 98(12): 2163–2171.
27. Odberg T, Riise D. Early diagnosis of glaucoma. II. The value of the initial examination in ocular hypertension. Acta Ophthalmol 1987; 65: 58.
28. de Voogd S, Ikram MK, Wolfs RC, Jansonius NM, Hofman A, de Jong PT. Incidence of open-angle glaucoma in a general elderly population: the Rotterdam Study. Ophthalmology 2005; 112: 1487–1493.
29. Armaly MF, Krueger DE, Maundir L, *et al*. Bio-statistical analysis of the Collaborative Glaucoma Study. I. Summary report of the risk factors for glaucomatous visual-field defects. Arch Ophthalmol 1980; 98: 2163–2171.
30. Klein BEK, Klein R, Sponsel WE, *et al*. Prevalence of glaucoma. The Beaver Dam Eye Study. Ophthalmology 1992; 99: 1499–1504.
31. David R, Tessler Z, Yassur Y. Epidemiology of acute angle closure glaucoma: incidence and seasonal variations. Ophthalmologica 1985; 191: 4–7.
32. Teikari J, Raivio I, Nurminen M. Incidence of acute glaucoma in Finland from 1973–1982. Graefe's Arch Clin Exp Ophthalmol 1987; 225: 357–360.
33. Congdon N, Wang F, Tielsch JM. Issues in the epidemiology and population-based screening of primary angle-closure glaucoma. Surv Ophthalmol 1992; 36: 411–423.
34. Martin MJ, Sommer A, Gold EB, *et al*. Race and primary open angle glaucoma. Am J Ophthalmol 1985; 99: 383–387.
35. The advanced glaucoma intervention study (AGIS). 3. Baseline characteristics of black and white patients. Ophthalmology 1998; 105: 1137–1145.
36. Quigley HA. Number of people with glaucoma worldwide. Br J Ophthalmol 1996; 80: 389–393.
37. Genio CA, Gavino BC. Glaucoma profile in the Philippines General Hospital. Philipp J Ophthalmol 1983; 15: 1–2.
38. Arkell SM, Lightman DA, Sommer A, *et al*. The prevalence of glaucoma among Eskimos of Northwest Alaska. Arch Ophthalmol 1987; 105: 482.
39. Sung VCT, Koppens JM, Vernon SA, Pawson P, Rubinstein M, King AJ and Tattersall CL. Longitudinal glaucoma screening for siblings of patients with primary open angle glaucoma: the Nottingham Family Glaucoma Screening Study. Br J Ophthalmol 2006; 90: 59–63.
40. Rosenthal AR, Perkins ES. Family studies in glaucoma. Br J Ophthalmol 1985; 69: 664–667.
41. Tielsch JM, Katz J, Sommer A, *et al*. Family history and risk of primary open angle glaucoma. The Baltimore Eye Survey. Arch Ophthalmol 1994; 112: 69–73.
42. Nemesure B, Leske MC, He Q, *et al*. Analyses of reported family history of glaucoma: a preliminary investigation. The Barbados Eye Study Group. Ophthalmic Epidemiol 1996; 3: 135–141.
43. Wu J, Hewitt AW, Green CM, Ring MA, McCartney PJ, Craig JE, Mackey DA. Disease severity of familial glaucoma compared with sporadic glaucoma. Arch Ophthalmol 2006; 124: 950–954.

44. Perkins ES, Phelps CD. Open-angle glaucoma, ocular hypertension, low-tension glaucoma, and refraction. Arch Ophthalmol 1982; 100: 1464–1467.
45. Daubs JG, Crick RP. Effect of refractive error on the risk of ocular hypertension and open-angle glaucoma. Trans Ophthalmol Soc 1981; 101: 121.
46. Mitchell P, Hourihan F, Sandbach J, Wang J. The relationship between glaucoma and myopia: The Blue Mountains Eye Study. Ophthalmology 1999; 106: 2010–2015.
47. Lotofo D, Ritch R, Szmyd L Jr, Burris JE. Juvenile glaucoma, race, and refraction. JAMA 1989; 261: 249–252.
48. Yamamoto T, Iwase A, Kawase K, Sawada A, Ishida K. Optic disc hemorrhages detected in a large-scale eye disease screening project. J Glaucoma 2004; 13: 356–360.
49. Kono Y, Sugiyama K, Ishida K, Yamamoto T, Kitazawa Y. Characteristics of visual field progression in patients with normal-tension glaucoma with optic disk hemorrhages. Am J Ophthalmol 2003; 135: 499–503.
50. Ahn JK, Park KH. Morphometric change analysis of the optic nerve head in unilateral disk hemorrhage cases. Am J Ophthalmol 2002; 134: 920–922.
51. Ishida K, Yamamoto T, Sugiyama K, Kitazawa Y. Disk hemorrhage is a significantly negative prognostic factor in normal-tension glaucoma. Am J Ophthalmol 2000; 129: 707–714.
52. Budenz DL, Anderson DR, Feuer WJ, Beiser JA, Schiffman J, Parrish RK 2nd, Piltz-Seymour JR, Gordon MO, Kass MA. Ocular Hypertension Treatment Study Group. Detection and Prognostic Significance of Optic Disc Hemorrhages during the Ocular Hypertension Treatment Study. Ophthalmology 2006 Sep 21 (Epub ahead of print).
52. Dielemans I, de Jong PT, Stolk R, *et al.* Primary open-angle glaucoma, intraocular pressure, and diabetes mellitus in the general elderly population. The Rotterdam Study. Ophthalmology 1996; 103(8): 1271–1275.
53. Klein BEK, Klein R, Jensen SC. Open-angle glaucoma and older-onset diabetes. The Beaver Dam Eye Study. Ophthalmology 1994; 101(7): 1173–1177.
54. Pasquale LR, Kang JH, Manson JE, Willett WC, Rosner BA, Hankinson SE. Prospective study of type 2 diabetes mellitus and risk of primary open-angle glaucoma in women. Ophthalmology 2006; 113: 1081–1086.
55. Kass MA, Heuer DK, Higginbotham EJ, Johnson CA, Keltner JL, Miller JP, Parrish RK 2nd, Wilson MR, Gordon MO. The Ocular Hypertension Treatment Study: a randomized trial determines that topical ocular hypotensive medication delays or prevents the onset of primary open-angle glaucoma. Arch Ophthalmol 2002; 120: 701–713.
56. Mitchell P, Smith W, Chey T, Healey PR. Open-angle glaucoma and diabetes: the Blue Mountain Eye Study, Australia. Ophthalmology 1997; 104(4): 712–718.
57. de Voogd S, Ikram MK, Wolfs RC, Jansonius NM, Witteman JC, Hofman A, de Jong PT. Is diabetes mellitus a risk factor for open-angle glaucoma? The Rotterdam Study. Ophthalmology 2006; 113: 1827–1831.
58. Langman MJ, Lancashire RJ, Cheng KK, Stewart PM. Systemic hypertension and glaucoma: mechanisms in common and co-occurrence. Br J Ophthalmol 2005; 89: 960–963.
59. Graham SL, Drance SM, Wijsman K, *et al.* Ambulatory blood pressure monitoring in glaucoma. The nocturnal dip. Ophthalmology 1995; 102(1): 61–69.
60. Smith KD, Arthurs BP, Saheb N. An association between hypothyroidism and primary open-angle glaucoma. Ophthalmology 1993; 100: 1580–1584.
61. Girkin CA, McGwin G Jr, McNeal SF, Lee PP, Owsley C. Hypothyroidism and the development of open-angle glaucoma in a male population. Ophthalmology 2004; 111: 1649–1652.
62. Phelps CD, Corbett JJ. Migraine and low-tension glaucoma: a case-control study. Invest Ophthalmol Vis Sci l985; 26: 1105.
63. Wang JJ, Mitchell P, Smith W. Is there an association between migraine headache and open-angle glaucoma? Findings from the Blue Mountains Eye Study. Ophthalmology 1997; 104: 1714–1719.

64. Klein BE, Klein R, Meuer SM, Goetz LA. Migraine headache and its association with open-angle glaucoma: the Beaver Dam Eye Study. Invest Ophthalmol Vis Sci 1993; 34: 3024–3027.
65. Usui T, Iwata K, Shirakashi M, Abe H. Prevalence of migraine in low-tension glaucoma and primary open-angle glaucoma in Japanese. Br J Ophthalmol 1991; 75: 224–226.
66. Anderson DR. Normal Tension Glaucoma Study. Collaborative normal tension glaucoma study. Curr Opin Ophthalmol 2003; 14: 86–90.
67. Cursiefen C, Wisse M, Cursiefen S, Junemann A, Martus P, Korth M. Migraine and tension headache in high-pressure and normal-pressure glaucoma. Am J Ophthalmol 2000;129: 102–104.

Chapter 3

Genetics

Why should I read this chapter?

It's short for a start! You will be seeing glaucoma patients day-in day-out and they will inevitably ask you whether their family members should be screened for glaucoma. Moreover when assessing glaucoma suspects you need to know whether their family history is truly significant and what implications it has for your patient. We cannot counsel our patients appropriately if we do not have a basic understanding of the genetics behind the disorder.

Genetics

It is clear that a significant risk factor for the development of glaucoma is a family history.[1–4] Naturally different sorts of glaucoma will have different inheritance patterns and the likelihood of getting the disease will be linked to the closeness of the family member afflicted. This likelihood is called the genetic risk and is generally greater for first-degree relatives such as parents and siblings (who share about 50% of the genetic material), lower for second-degree relatives such as aunts, uncles and grandparents (who share approx 25% of the patient's genetic material), and lowest for third-degree relatives such as first cousins (who share 12.5%).

Primary open-angle glaucoma: adult onset

Glaucoma occurring in adults is generally inherited in a multifactorial manner.[1,3] It is not a clear-cut issue and thus if both parents have glaucoma it is not certain that the child will inevitably develop glaucoma in later life. Their risk will be increased but it is the combination of multiple genetic factors and environmental factors which will trigger the disease. If that, currently incompletely understood, group of factors does not manifest then the patient will be spared.

To date, at least 20 genetic loci for POAG have been reported.[5] Only three causative genes are identified from these loci: myocilin (MYOC), optineurin (OPTN) and WD repeat domain 36 (WDR36). Despite the excitement about these 'glaucoma' genes, mutations in them have only been found in less than 10% of patients with POAG.[5–7] Only one of these specific genes, the TIGR/Myocilin gene (MYOC), has been shown to confer definite susceptibility to adult-onset POAG[5] and the presence of a mutation in this gene in an affected patient puts the risk to first-degree family members as high as 50%.[8,9]

Juvenile-onset open-angle glaucoma

This disorder usually has autosomal dominant inheritance and thus, on average, 50% of members of any generation of the family are affected with equal sex predeliction. Mutations in MYOC have been shown to be responsible for up to one quarter of cases of juvenile open-angle glaucoma.[6,7,10]

Primary congenital glaucoma

Congenital glaucoma is frequently inherited as an autosomal recessive trait but can also be sporadic in nature. Carriers of the defective gene are asymptomatic and only when both of them pass this gene on to their offspring does the disease manifest. This can occur more frequently within cultures where consanguinity is common. The risk to the brother or sister of a child with congenital glaucoma is in the region of 25%.

Axenfeld-Rieger syndrome

This is one of the anterior segment dysgenesis syndromes. These encompass a spectrum of developmental disorders resulting in abnormal formation of the structures of the anterior segment. About half of those affected develop glaucoma due to malformation of the aqueous outflow mechanisms of the eye. They tend be be inherited in an autosomal dominant fashion so they are passed almost directly down the family tree. This may not be obvious as there is massive variability in the expression of the resulting defect. For example one individual may have a marked abnormality and develop severe glaucoma while their offspring may have minimal changes and never develop raised IOP. First-degree relatives of an individual with an anterior segment dysgenesis syndrome have a 50:50 chance of developing the syndrome and, if they do have it, a subsequent 50% chance of getting glaucoma. In patients who do have these syndromes there is no way to predict which ones will develop glaucoma, although obviously those with excessive morphological abnormalities in the drainage angle are likely suspects for future raised IOP.

Pigment dispersion syndrome and pigmentary glaucoma

The pigment dispersion syndrome may be inherited in an autosomal dominant fashion although there are many sporadic cases seen in clinical practice. About half of all individuals with pigment dispersion will develop pigmentary glaucoma.[11] Again it is impossible to predict which of those patients with this syndrome will go on to develop raised IOP. First-degree relatives of affected individuals have a 50:50 chance of developing it themselves.

Aniridia

Mutations in the PAX6 gene cause aniridia, a developmental disorder which results in anterior segment dysgenesis. The inheritance is autosomal dominant and first-degree relatives have a

50% chance of inheriting the disease. Some of these patients go on to develop glaucoma. Glaucoma may be present in about a third of cases and is often the main cause of visual loss.[12]

References

1. Wolfs RC, Klaver CC, Ramrattan RS, *et al.* Genetic risk of primary open-angle glaucoma: Population-based familial aggregation study. Arch Ophthalmol 1998; 116: 1640–1645.
2. Tielsch JM, Katz J, Sommer A, *et al.* Family history and risk of primary open angle glaucoma. The Baltimore Eye Survey. Arch Ophthalmol 1994; 112: 69–73.
3. Nemesure B, He Q, Mendell N, *et al.* Inheritance of open-angle glaucoma in the Barbados Family Study Am J Med Genet 2001; 103: 36–43.
4. Sung VCT, Koppens JM, Vernon SA, Pawson P, Rubinstein M, King AJ, Tattersall CL. Longitudinal glaucoma screening for siblings of patients with primary open angle glaucoma: the Nottingham Family Glaucoma Screening Study. Br J Ophthalmol 2006; 90: 59–63.
5. Fan BJ, Wang DY, Lam DS, Pang CP. Gene mapping for primary open angle glaucoma. Clin Biochem 2006; 39: 249–258.
6. Wiggs JL, Allingham RR, Vollrath D, *et al.* Prevalence of mutations in TIGR/Myocilin in patients with adult and juvenile primary open-angle glaucoma. Am J Hum Genet 1998; 63: 1549–1552.
7. Fingert JH, Heon E, Liebmann JM, *et al.* Analysis of myocilin mutations in 1,703 glaucoma patients from five different populations. Hum Mol Genet 1999; 8: 899–905.
8. Allingham RR, Wiggs JL, De La Paz MA, *et al.* Gln368STOP myocilin mutation in families with late-onset primary open-angle glaucoma. Invest Ophthalmol Vis Sci 1998; 39: 2288–2295.
9. Craig JE, Barid PN, Healey DL, *et al.* Evidence for genetic heterogeneity within eight glaucoma families, with the GLC1A Gln368STOP mutation being a important phenotypic modifier. Ophthalmology 2001; 108: 1607–1620.
10. Adam MF, Belmouden A, Binisti P, *et al.* Recurrent mutations in a single exon encoding the evolutionarily conserved olfactomedin-homology domain of TIGR in familial open-angle glaucoma. Hum Mol Genet 1997; 6: 2091–2097.
11. Ritch R. Pigment Dispersion Syndrome. Am J Opthhalmology 1998; 126: 425–431.
12. Valenzuela A, Cline RA. Ocular and nonocular findings in patients with aniridia. Can J Ophthalmol 2004; 39: 632–638.

Chapter 4

The pathophysiology of glaucoma

Why should I read this chapter?

It is important to understand a little of how and why glaucoma happens. This chapter is purposefully short and does not go into depth about the exact pathophysiology of glaucoma. There are massive textbooks which spend dozens of pages addressing this issue and the literature is packed with scientific data on this subject. It is not possible to leave out this issue entirely as some of the concepts and ideas will have implications on how and why our management works.

Introduction

Elevated intraocular pressure (IOP) is a risk factor for developing glaucomatous damage to the optic nerve. Despite a lack of complete understanding of the exact mechanisms involved it is clear that the link between raised IOP and glaucoma is probably causal.[1] IOP is not, however, the be-all and end-all of glaucoma. Some patients may develop features of glaucoma with a normal IOP and others may have a significantly elevated IOP and develop no glaucoma whatsoever.

Despite vast amounts of laboratory and clinical research the exact etiology of glaucomatous optic neuropathy remains uncertain. We know that ganglion cell axons are dying at the level of the lamina cribrosa with retrograde atrophy back to their cell bodies in the retina. Glaucomatous optic nerve damage is inevitably due to a variety or combination of pathogenic factors.

Factors that may play a role in pathogenesis are:

- Elevated IOP
- Poor vascular perfusion pressure to the ONH
- Intermittent ONH ischemia
- Mechanical compression of ganglion cell axons at the scleral ring
- Obstruction of axoplasmic flow within the ganglion cell axon
- Excessive pressure-dependent movement of potentially weakened lamina cribrosa
- Faulty connective tissue support for nerve fibers at the lamina cribrosa

- Release of excitotoxins in the optic nerve
- Induction of programmed cell death of the ganglion cell axons (apoptosis)

Intraocular pressure damage mechanisms

The defining phenomenon underlying glaucomatous optic neuropathy is damage to the neural and connective tissues of the ONH. This damage manifests clinically as ONH cupping, nerve fiber loss and visual-field defects. Presumably IOP-related connective tissue stress and strain, in addition to IOP-mediated ONH hypoperfusion, lead to cell loss with consequent posterior deformation and excavation of the ONH surface. Concurrent glaucomatous visual-field loss occurs as a result with development of visual morbidity.

Why should some nerves survive in complete health with IOPs of 28 mmHg while others experience significant glaucoma damage with IOPs of 20 mmHg? No-one knows the exact reason. Different eyes behave differently and there must be some specific relationship between the way any given IOP load is distributed amongst the load-bearing components of the eye, including the scleral shell and lamina cribrosa, as well as the overlying neural tissue. This relationship is individualized to a specific eye as is the response to alleviating this load by decreasing IOP.

Whatever the critical level of IOP at which an eye starts to become damaged it is clear that the laminar and prelaminar axonal nutrient supply is compromised. This degree of compromise may be exacerbated by IOP fluctuations, as consequent movement (or bounce) of the lamina cribrosa in response to the changing stresses may 'pinch' axons as they traverse this critical region.

A certain amount of potential structural damage at the level of the ONH may or may not result in axonal damage. Different nerves will respond differently to the pathophysiologic stresses induced by whichever mechanism, or combination of mechanisms, is actually occurring.

Vascular pathology

The link between vascular dysregulation in NTG is becoming better characterized; there is evidence to suggest that systemic autonomic failure and ocular vascular malfunction also occur in POAG patients.[2]

Why does the IOP go up?

There are several different causes, however a common theme with all the conditions is the fact that aqueous outflow cannot keep up with aqueous inflow. Therefore the fine balance is interrupted and IOP goes up. In patients with primary and secondary closed-angle glaucoma the reason for the aqueous outflow obstruction is apparent. In secondary open-angle glaucoma we can understand the reason for the blockage and clogging of the sieve-like trabecular meshwork. In primary open-angle glaucoma the exact pathogenesis is still not fully understood, however we do know that there is resistance at the cellular level in the juxtacanalicular trabecular meshwork.

References

1. Bahrami H. Causal inference in primary open angle glaucoma: specific discussion on intraocular pressure. Ophthalmic Epidemiol 2006; 13: 283–289.
2. Gherghel D, Hosking SL, Cunliffe IA. Abnormal systemic and ocular vascular response to temperature provocation in primary open-angle glaucoma patients: a case for autonomic failure? Invest Ophthalmol Vis Sci 2004; 45: 3546–3554.

Chapter 5

Anterior segment examination

Why should I read this chapter?

Examination of the patient is of course paramount to making a diagnosis of glaucoma but an accurate history can also give you valuable clues as to what is going on. Detecting raised IOP with a cupped disc and a visual field consistent with a glaucomatous optic neuropathy is not the end of your diagnostic examination. Unfortunately, the diagnosis is frequently not so clear-cut and that is where we earn our money. You need now to undertake a thorough examination to determine what form of glaucoma it is. Is it primary or secondary to another pathology? Is it normal tension or is the angle occluded or occludable? These factors will have a massive implication on how you treat your patient and will allow you to make long-term management plans. Erroneous initial diagnosis will lead to significant problems in the long run. This chapter will explain the *minimum* requirements for an examination of the anterior segment.

Introduction

Jumping to the examination will miss an awful lot of valuable and often essential information. A thorough history is vital before any examination commences. When first presented with a patient who may have glaucoma it is necessary to take a full history including their past medical history, their past ophthalmic history, any medication they take, any allergies they have, their social circumstances and family history. Even if the patient is known to have glaucoma and they are transferred to your care it is important to start again and go through the history. Not only may you elicit something which has been missed previously but you may also get an idea of the course of the patient's glaucoma management. For example; if they have had a previous trabeculectomy which failed after a week it has significant implications for future surgical interventions. If they had a good response to SLT in the past then this may remain a viable option for future IOP lowering.

The first examination is never a glaucoma examination. It is a general ophthalmic examination and requires thorough attention to the anterior and posterior segments as well as the lids and the periocular skin. Although the focus is naturally aimed at confirming or refuting a diagnosis of glaucoma it is vital that ocular comorbidity is not inadvertently missed. Loss of vision attributed to glaucoma progression may be actually due to a maculopathy, lens opacity or corneal pathology. A field defect thought to represent glaucoma may be a congenital defect, a manifestation of a retinal scar or a retinal detachment, or related to a tilted disc or disc drusen. Even more worrying is that the patient may have a space-occupying lesion causing the field defect.

The patient is attending an eye care professional and thus we have a duty of care to give them a thorough examination. In addition, any ocular comorbidity may have significant implications on further treatment of their glaucoma.

History

Presenting complaint

Why is the patient with you? How did they get there? Did they present because of symptoms or was this an incidental finding of a routine optometric visit?

Symptoms may have significant bearing on the diagnosis or they may be a red herring. Often when a patient is informed that they will be referred because of a suspicion of glaucoma they concentrate more upon their ocular status and will dredge up symptoms such as heaviness, occasional pain or intermittent blurring. These may be erroneous and insignificant but the clinician should be on the look out for red flags. The headache and nausea that occur in the evening associated with blurred vision and a red eye may be a hallmark of intermittent angle-closure attacks. Loss of central acuity may be the presenting feature of end-stage glaucoma. Halos may be features of transient corneal edema or related to pigmentary glaucomas (often occurring just after exercising) or uveitic problems such as Posner Schlossman syndrome.

POAG is usually painless unless the IOP is massively raised or there are rapid fluctuations in pressure. Concurrent intraocular inflammation may result in pain or photophobia. Ocular pain is usually described as an ache in the eye but may be localized to the brow. If the pain is associated with watering the pressure may have increased enough to cause corneal edema.

Past medical history

You have to know about your patients' past medical history. They may have other conditions which are risk factors for glaucoma (see Chapter 2) or they may have other problems which would have implications on your management. If a patient has metastatic breast cancer then you need to know this in case the optic nerve is being compressed by a metastasis or the patient's prognosis for survival is limited and aggressive interventions may be inappropriate. If the patient has severe rheumatoid arthritis they may have difficulties administering their drops. If they had a previous severe injury there may be an optic neuropathy secondary to severe blood loss. The eye can be affected by innumerable systemic disorders and thus it is important to elicit these. Ask about Raynaud's and migraine as they are important when assessing a potential normal-tension glaucoma patient.

Family history

Does anyone in the family have glaucoma or are there any other ocular conditions that may run in the family?

Past ocular history

Has the patient had any previous ocular problems? Have they been previously assessed for glaucoma? Scrutinizing the findings of that time may give an indication as to whether things have changed. Reliable documentation that a disc had no cup 5 years ago and now has a 0.7 cup-to-disc ratio is compelling evidence that things are changing and they do indeed have glaucoma.

Has the patient had any previous surgery to the eye? Has there ever been any previous intra-ocular inflammation? Recurrent episodes of iritis may result in eventual synechial angle closure with subsequent secondary ACG. Prolonged topical steroid used to treat recurrent uveitis may have played a part in the pathogenesis of a new glaucoma.

Has there been any previous history of trauma? Previous significant blunt injury may have resulted in angle damage resulting in angle-recession glaucoma many years later.

Social history

Who is at home with the patient? Will they have someone to put drops in if they need to be treated? What sort of family support structure is available to ensure compliance with prescribed medication? There is nothing like a nagging wife to ensure compliance in a patient (author's personal communication).

Smoking and alcohol are not directly linked to glaucoma although alcoholism and subsequent vitamin deficiency can result in visual loss. When considering a problem of ONH perfusion it makes sense to maximize the amount of oxygen in the bloodstream, and therefore for that reason (amongst hundreds of other) it is sensible to advise our glaucoma patients to stop smoking.

Medications

What tablets does the patient take? Some medications may cause pupil dilatation and may precipitate angle-closure episodes. Some medications may cause retinal toxicity directly. Anticoagulants such as warfarin and aspirin may have significant implications if surgery is planned.

Nocturnal anti-hypertensives may play a part in overnight dips in blood pressure and subsequent worsening of glaucoma, particularly NTG.

Summary

The above may seem excessively laborious but such a detailed assessment will usually only have to be undertaken once when the patient is first referred to your care. Such baseline information will help with diagnosis and aid in devising a patient-specific individualized management plan. Asking the patient periodically during their follow-up whether anything has changed is prudent.

Examination techniques

Visual acuity

Examination should begin with an accurate assessment of visual acuity. An accurate up-to-date refraction is helpful however pin-hole acuity should suffice to suggest visual potential.

Pupil reactions

The main reason to examine the pupil reactions is to assess for the presence of a relative afferent papillary defect (RAPD). This may suggest severe asymmetric optic nerve pathology. It is important to appreciate that it is a comparative test and will compare function between the two eyes. If the patient has equal disease in both eyes there will be no detectable RAPD. If one eye has much more advanced glaucoma than the other an RAPD may be detected.

Slit lamp examination

Lids

Have a quick look at the lids for evidence of any skin pathology, signs of allergic problems (potentially related to prolonged use of glaucoma drops) and blepharitis which may have implications in the presence of a failing trabeculectomy bleb.

Conjunctiva

In most cases the conjunctiva will often be normal.

Look for conjunctival scarring. Although this may not have a direct implication on their current status, if future surgical intervention is required it will be of paramount importance. This is best accomplished by moving the anesthetized conjunctiva with a cotton-tipped applicator, but may be grossly assessed by moving the upper lid over the conjunctiva and watching for free movement.

Look for redness. Acute angle closure or uveitis will result in redness and ciliary injection. Mild conjunctival hyperemia may occur with chronic use of medications, particularly prostaglandin analogs. Conjunctival injection with a follicular reaction is commonly seen as a sign of topical drug hypersensitivity.

Look at the episcleral vasculature. Dilated episcleral vessels in an otherwise quiet eye suggest increased episcleral venous pressure. These vessels appear 'beefy', straighter and are radially orientated. Assessing redness and conjunctival vascular engorgement has a vital role to play in the management of post-glaucoma surgery patients.

Look for abnormal areas of sclera. Thin areas of sclera should be identified, as future therapy in the form of surgery or cyclodiode laser will need to avoid these areas.

Cornea

Look for corneal edema. Markedly raised IOP will result in epithelial edema and bullae. There are numerous other causes of corneal edema which must be considered and excluded. If the IOP is normal a primary corneal pathology must be suspected.

Look at the corneal endothelium. In young people with unilateral glaucoma watch out for endothelial changes and edema consistent with iridocorneal endothelial (ICE) syndrome. The classical pigment vertical spindle will be seen in pigmentary dispersion syndrome (PDS) (Fig. 5.1) or sometimes in pseudoexfoliation (PXE). Keratic precipitates can suggest active or past uveitis (Fig. 5.2). With extensive PXE, white flakes themselves may be found on the endothelial surface.

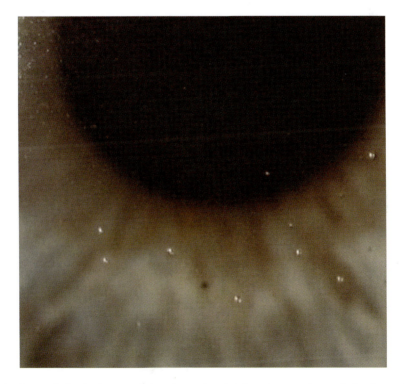

Figure 5.1 Krukenberg spindle. A close-up of the cornea showing the presence of a vertical column of pigmentation on the endothelium characteristic of a Krukenberg spindle.

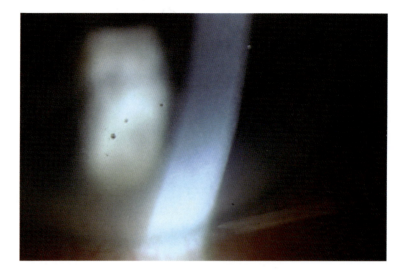

Figure 5.2 Keratic precipitates. A close-up of the inferior cornea showing the presence of fine white new keratic precipitates and older and larger pigmented ones.

Measure CCT. Given the ease of CCT measurement it is reasonable to measure it in every new patient. The influence on management in established glaucoma is equivocal but in ocular hypertensive patients its assessment is mandatory (see Chapter 10).

Anterior chamber

Assess the depth of the AC. Make a conscious effort to evaluate and document central and peripheral AC depth. Using a thin slit look at the anterior surface of the lens and focus yourself on the distance to the posterior surface of the cornea. Experience will allow you to immediately judge which ACs are deep and which are shallow. Once you are happy with your assessment of the central AC move to the peripheral cornea and re-assess the depth there. Reasonably deep central ACs can shallow rapidly towards the peripheries. The angle needs to be assessed formally and warrants a separate chapter in its own right (see Chapter 6).

Iris

Iris changes may be associated with an underlying pathology or may be due to the elevated IOP.

Look for different colored irides. Differences in the color of the iris between eyes (heterochromia) may occur in heterochromic iridocyclitis (Fig. 5.3). The lighter iris is usually the pathological eye as the iris stroma atrophies and allows the iris pigment layer to manifest in the iris color. Sometimes unilateral prostaglandin use will result in different color irides.

Look for PXE: white flecks may be seen at the pupillary ruff (Fig. 5.4).

Look for abnormal vessels. Use high magnification to spot the fine tufts of neovascular vessels (Fig. 5.5) which can occur at the pupillary margin in neovascular glaucoma. Normal iris blood

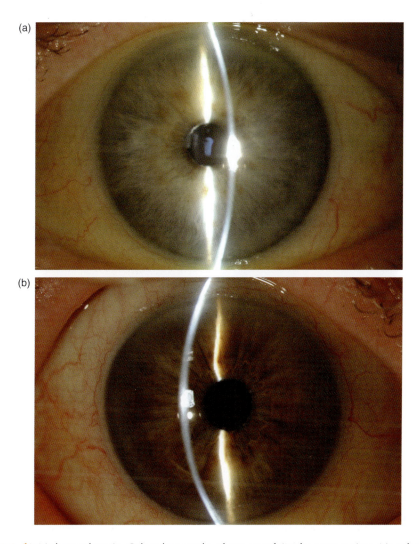

Figure 5.3 (a) & (b) Iris heterochromia. Color photographs of two eyes from the same patient. Iris color is markedly different between the eyes.

vessels are radial but distinction between normal and pathological vessels can be difficult in inflamed eyes when the native vasculature is engorged.

Look for localized atrophy. Sector iris atrophy is typical in herpes zoster ophthalmicus uveitis. Atrophy in the iridocorneal endothelial (ICE) syndrome may eventually lead to hole formation with accompanying corectopia (Fig. 5.6) and ectropion uveae. Nodules may also occur in the Cogan-Reese variant of ICE. Repeated episodes of markedly raised IOP may result in several areas of atrophy.

Look for iris transillumination defects. Switch the room lights off and narrow the slit vertically until it fits into the pupil. Line it up down the visual axis and look at the red reflex. In normal eyes no red reflex will be seen through the iris. Peripupillary defects are frequently observed in PXE. Midperiphery radial slits are seen in PDS (Fig. 5.7).

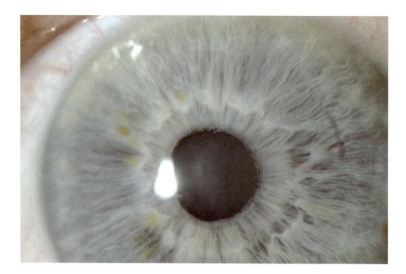

Figure 5.4 Pseudoexfoliation – pupillary fibrillary matter. Color photograph with fine fibrillary pseudoexfoliative matter at the pupil margin.

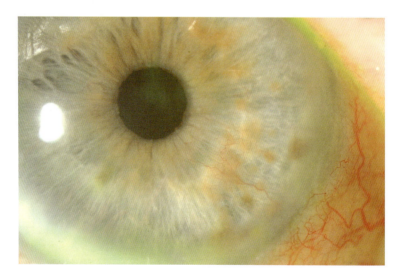

Figure 5.5 Neovascular vessels. Color photograph of the iris showing extensive irregular branching new vessels.

Lens

Look for a cataract. The patient may have a visually significant cataract. This may be the main cause of their acuity loss or may be the reason why their visual fields are unreliable. In addition if glaucoma surgery is contemplated, the surgeon may elect to proceed to cataract surgery first and then glaucoma surgery or they may decide to undertake a combined procedure. Significant cataract can cause forward displacement of the iris due to an increase in its axial dimensions.

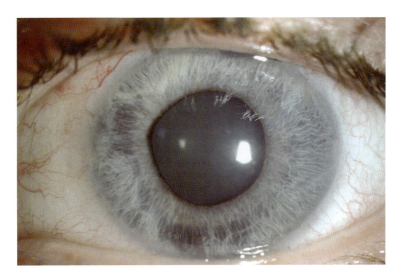

Figure 5.6 Corectopia in iridocorneal endothelial syndrome. Color photograph showing early ICE syndrome with mild distortion of pupil shape (corectopia). (Courtesy of Mr A.J. King)

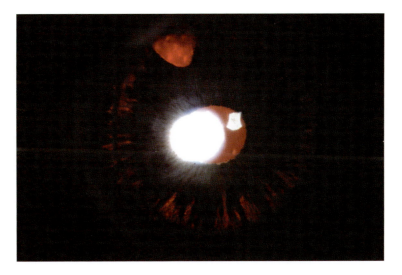

Figure 5.7 Advanced pigment dispersion syndrome with spoke-like iris transillumination defects. The patient has had a trabeculectomy and a peripheral iridotomy is visible superiorly.

This can cause a form of AAC called phacomorphic glaucoma. Compare to the other eye to see whether the AC is significantly shallower due to the mature cataract.

Look for evidence of previous inflammation. Look for posterior synechiae or pigment on the lens surface.

Look for PXE. Look for the white flaky material on the lens surface (usually in the classical three zones) (Fig. 5.8).

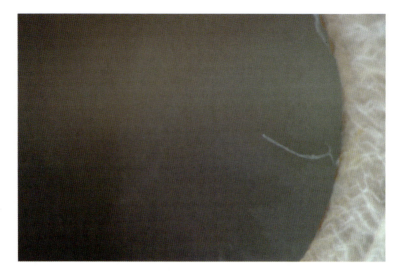

Figure 5.8 Pseudoexfoliation – three zones. Color photograph focused on the anterior lens surface. A central zone of white material is seen on the anterior lens bordered by a clear zone where the pupil has rubbed this material off. Finally there is a further outer zone of pseudoexfoliative material.

Look at the position of the lens. Is it central? Is it displaced vertically, horizontally or anteriorly? Is it mobile? Often tapping the slit lamp firmly with your knuckles can create enough movement to cause the lens to 'wobble' if it is unstable (phacodonesis). This may occur in certain congenital disorders, after trauma or in severe PXE and may result in pupillary block.

Look for glaucomflecken. These are bubbles in the anterior lens substance related to previous episodes of markedly raised IOP.

Gonioscopy

All patients should have gonioscopy when they first attend the eye service as a matter of routine (see Chapter 6).

To dilate or not to dilate – that is the question

In the great majority of patients there will be no problem with dilating them with a short-acting mydriatic such as tropicamide (1%). A clear view of the posterior pole is vital to complete the ophthalmic examination and also to assess the disc correctly. *It is impossible to get a true clear stereo impression of the optic disc without a dilated pupil.* You can make best guesses as to the state of the ONH, and indeed the majority of follow-ups will be undertaken relying on examination with an undilated pupil, but in order to get a true assessment and to look for subtle thinning of the neuroretinal rim, optic disc hemorrhages and nerve fiber layer defects the patient will have to be dilated. The concern is the induction of AAC.

If a patient has sustained a previous attack of AAC and they have not received any prophylactic measures to prevent a further attack (such as a surgical or laser peripheral iridotomy) then it is prudent not to dilate them until this is done.

If you examine the AC and note that it is shallow peripherally then you need to formally assess the angle to decide whether it is occludable. If you decide that it is occludable then prophylactic laser peripheral iridotomies may be indicated before dilatation. In some situations even if the angle looks occludable you can dilate safely. Pharmacological drops take the pupil through the dangerous mid-dilated phase very quickly and thus pupil block and AAC may not develop even in predisposed eyes (see Chapter 22). The more worrying time is when the pupil slowly returns to normal and patients should be warned about the symptoms of AAC and advised to reattend should they experience them. Another argument may be that iatrogenic induction of AAC may not be a bad thing and that stimulating an event that would have happened eventually anyway is a good thing – effectively using it as a diagnostic provocation test. If such patients are dilated the IOP should be rechecked again and the patient warned that if they develop redness, reduced vision and pain they need to attend the hospital eye service for potential treatment. Just because someone has safely dilated the pupil without an IOP rise does not necessarily mean that they do not have potentially occludable angles.

Chapter 6

Assessing the angle

Why should I read this chapter?

You cannot manage a glaucoma patient without being able to assess the angle. Glaucoma is about pressure and you cannot escape the fact that without knowing whether the drainage system is morphologically intact you cannot speculate as to the cause for any raised IOP and thus intuitively you cannot hope to treat it adequately. You need to assess the angle initially by the van Herrick technique then by formal gonioscopy. Gonioscopy is not easy and only practice will allow you to become competent.

Introduction

Assessment of the drainage angle is a vital step in the initial assessment of a glaucoma patient. If the situation changes with the passage of time there may be a need to repeat it but usually once the angle is documented as being open there is no need to repeat it with any significant frequency.

There are two main methods used to examine the drainage angle; the van Herrick technique and gonioscopy. Gonioscopy remains the gold standard method and its routine use should be encouraged.

van Herrick technique

The van Herrick technique[1] has proven to be a useful tool in the assessment of the AC angle.

The patient is sat at the slit lamp and asked to look forward. The slit lamp beam is placed at full intensity and narrowed as much as possible. It is placed at 60° off axial and then shone at the temporal limbus as far out as possible but still just within clear cornea. Increase the magnification and concentrate on the slit. Observe the thickness of the cornea and then focus your attention on the gap between the back of the cornea and the surface of the iris (the very peripheral anterior chamber depth). Compare the distance between corneal endothelium and iris surface to the overall thickness of the cornea to get a ratio (Fig. 6.1 and Table 6.1). It is

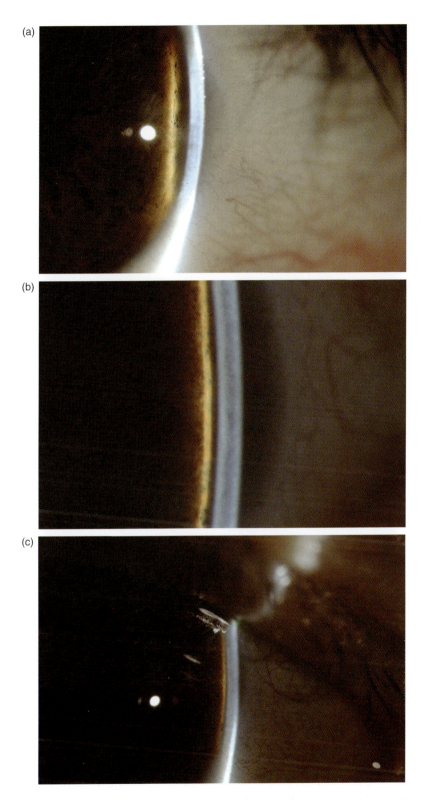

Figure 6.1 van Herricks of different depths. (a) Gap (much) thicker than one half thickness of cornea. This angle is wide open. (b) Gap thicker than one quarter thickness of cornea but less than half. This angle is open and not occludable. (c) Gap less than one quarter thickness of the cornea. This represents a narrow angle with a potential risk of angle closure.

Table 6.1 The van Herrick grading scheme.

Width of peripheral AC compared to corneal thickness	Equivalent Shaffer angle classification	What it means
>1/2 (gap thicker than one half thickness of cornea)	4	Angle wide open – not occludable
1/4 to 1/2 (gap thicker than one quarter thickness of cornea but less than half)	3	Reasonably open angle – not occludable
=1/4 (gap equals one quarter thickness of cornea)	2	Reasonably narrow angle – occlusion unlikely but possible
<1/4 (gap less than one quarter thickness of cornea)	1	Narrow angle – occludable, risk of angle closure
No clear gap or only slit size gap between cornea and iris	0	Very narrow angle – high risk of occlusion/angle closure or already in angle closure

important that the beam is as far out as possible, as having the beam too central may miss a narrow angle (Fig. 6.2).

A recent study[2] looked at almost 15000 patients finding good correlation between the van Herrick technique and the Shaffer grading by formal gonioscopy (see later).

Gonioscopy

Gonioscopy is the examination of the drainage angle utilizing a contact lens and biomicroscopy. It is vital that the angle is assessed before any management plans are made about a patient's glaucoma. Determination of the type of glaucoma and the mechanism of aqueous outflow obstruction cannot be done until the angle is formally visualized. Accurate gonioscopic evaluation of the iridocorneal angle is indispensable in allowing accurate diagnosis, classification, and management of glaucoma.

Gonioscopy should be done in every new patient. You may pick up something new or you may detect peripheral anterior synechiae (PAS) which have developed over the duration of their follow-up, potentially years after their initial presentation to an eye service. In patients who have sustained a central retinal vein occlusion, gonioscopy should be carried out monthly for the first 3 months to detect any evidence of early neovascularization.

Is there any point in doing gonioscopy in a patient with an IOP within the normal range? The answer is yes. It may seem like a pointless exercise, however it is still an important step. Patients who go on to develop synechial angle-closure glaucoma must start somewhere. Before the IOP rises they must develop some degree of progressive closure until they pass a certain threshold and the IOP goes up. This can be detected by gonioscopy and intervention considered. An IOP within the normal range at one measurement may be spiking to a much higher level at other times of the day. A patient with intermittent angle-closure glaucoma may have normal pressures when they are with you but be experiencing episodes of acutely raised IOP which can cause optic nerve compromise. Hence gonioscopy remains vital even in the presence of a normal IOP.

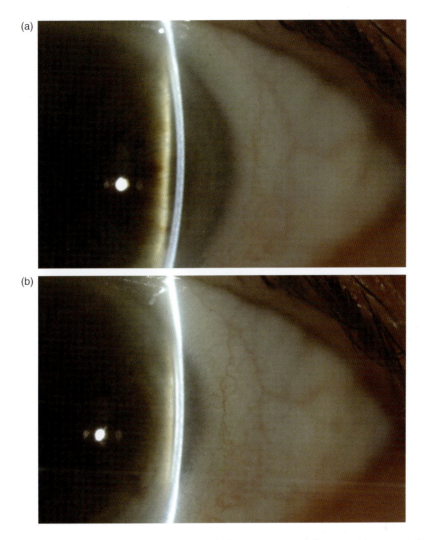

Figure 6.2 van Herrick technique. (a) Erroneously putting the beam too central shows a wide open angle. (b) Correct placement of the slit reveals a narrow angle.

Before gonioscopy is undertaken it is important to know what the examiner is looking for and thus an understanding of angle anatomy is required.

Angle anatomy

The AC angle is the area between the peripheral anterior iris insertion and the posterior surface of the peripheral cornea, marked anatomically as Schwalbe's line (Fig. 6.3). The primary

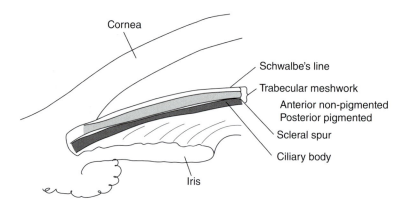

Figure 6.3 Diagram showing angle anatomy.

physiological function of the angle is to drain aqueous from the AC by filtering it through the trabecular meshwork into Schlemm's canal.

The visibility of structures seen at gonioscopy depends upon the concavity of the iris, its peripheral insertion point, and the depth of the angle. Essentially (and intuitively) the wider the angle the better view you will get. It is sensible to scrutinize angle anatomy by identifying the most posterior structure visible.

Ciliary body (CB)

The insertion of the iris root is usually into the anterior portion of the CB. The CB is only visible if the angle is widely open and may not be seen if the iris inserts more anteriorly. It is seen as a brown–grey-colored circumferential strip running around the whole angle. Color is variable according to race and may be darker in certain pathological conditions. Its width may be uneven depending upon where the iris inserts but if it is wider compared to the trabecular meshwork then angle recession must be suspected (see below). Occasionally, radially oriented normal blood vessels may be seen in the CB. These should not be confused with pathological neovascularization, which grows haphazardly from the surface of the iris across the ciliary body and scleral spur and over the trabecular meshwork.

PAS may cause localized or circumferential narrowing resulting in total obscuration of the CB.

Scleral spur

Immediately anterior to the CB is the white band of the scleral spur. This is usually the most easily identified landmark in the angle as it is bright white in stark contrast to the other pigmented structures. It lies directly between the trabecular meshwork and the CB.

Trabecular meshwork (TM)

This is why you look at the angle. The great majority of aqueous outflow occurs through the TM. If it is occluded the pressure will go up and the patient will eventually develop glaucoma. It is formed by three anatomically distinct portions. The uveal meshwork is the most central area and is comprised of a loose, lacy syncytium of connective tissue strands lined by endothelial cells. It usually covers the angle structures from the iris root to Schwalbe's line. The next layer out is the corneoscleral TM and is literally a mesh of connective tissue with holes and gaps that get progressively smaller as it moves closer to Schlemm's canal. The juxtacanalicular tissue is the outermost portion of the TM and lies immediately next to Schlemm's canal; it is this area which provides greatest resistance to aqueous outflow. It is thought that increased resistance in this layer causes the IOP to increase in POAG. The filtering TM stops pigment and other debris from entering the Schlemm's canal.

The anterior one half to one third of the TM is non-pigmented while the posterior more functional zone is variably pigmented.

Schwalbe's line (SL)

Just anterior to the non-pigmented area of the TM is SL. This is the most anterior structure seen in the angle and represents the end of Descemet's membrane. SL is a slightly elevated circumferential whitish, glistening ridge extending from the posterior surface of the cornea. It may occasionally be pigmented in pathological conditions.

When faced with a narrow angle or a markedly depigmented angle with anatomy hard to define, the identification of SL can be a vital tool. In order to identify the SL, narrow the slit down and tilt it slightly. Light from the narrow beam will now reflect off the anterior and posterior surface of the cornea. The two lines will meet at Schwalbe's line. Once Schwalbe's line is identified, every structure you can see posterior to it represents structures visible in an open angle.

The technique

The most common gonioscopic lenses in modern use are the Volk, Zeiss and Goldmann lenses. Each has pros and cons and often which is used is dependent upon personal preference. Purchase one and get on and use it on every patient and it should become second nature. The Goldmann is probably techinically easier to use for the beginner goinioscopist however the Zeiss or Volk four-mirror lenses tend to be used by glaucoma specialists.

The angle cannot be visualized directly due to total internal reflection of light by the peripheral cornea. Gonioscopy employs various contact lenses incorporating mirrors orientated to provide a view of the iridocorneal angle using reflected light. Examination is performed at the slit lamp biomicroscope.

The cornea should be anesthetized with a topical drop and a simple explanation offered to the patient to put them at ease. IOP should be measured prior to gonioscopy, as gonioscopy can have an massaging effect and artificially lower the readings obtained.

The Goldmann lens has a diameter which is greater than the cornea and a concave surface that is steeper than it. Its surface is not in contact with the cornea without the use of a coupling agent (such as Viscotears). The corneal curve of the lens is filled with the viscous solution and then the patient is asked to look up. Hold the lower lid down and apply the lens to the eye. Once the patient returns their gaze to the primary position the lens will center on the cornea. Because of its concave surface a suction effect is created helping maintain centration of the lens. This also allows the examiner to stabilize the globe and move the eye if required during examination or laser.

The other lenses (Zeiss and Volk) have a contact area which is smaller than the cornea and a shallower concavity. They do not need a coupling agent and will maintain contact with the cornea by gentle pressure using the native tear film as a coupling agent. When applying these lenses again ask the patient to look up to the ceiling, hold the lower lid and apply the lens gently (Fig. 6.4). It will not center by itself and the examiner needs to maintain its position on the cornea. Watch the tear film and ensure that contact is maintained across the whole surface of the lens throughout the examination.

Once the lens is applied offer reassurance to the patient and ask them to keep staring straight ahead, fixing on a point over your opposite shoulder. Line the slit beam up axially with the mirror you're looking at and broaden it slightly so you can get a good view of the angle.

IMPORTANT: The room lights must be off and the slit lamp beam as slim as possible. You need to prevent light getting into the pupil or you will induce pupil constriction and may artificially open the angle (it will be like having the patient on pilocarpine). This is a catch-22 as you need enough light to see what you need to but not enough to cause the pupil to constrict excessively. The examination must be of the physiological state of the angle in 'dusk' type illumination.

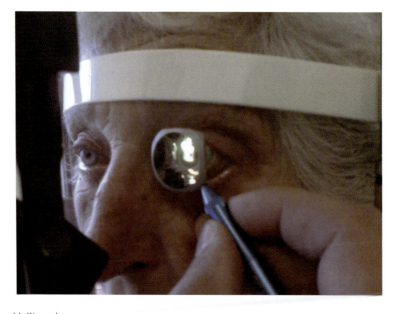

Figure 6.4 Use of lollipop lens.

Some of the Goldmann lenses only have one mirror and in order to examine the whole angle the lens will have to be rotated through 360° while moving the light of the slit lamp around, maintaining alignment on the mirror. With the four-mirror lenses you can leave the lens in place and look at the four portions of the angle simultaneously by moving the slit lamp. Remember that the structure under view is opposite the mirror.

You can move the lens slightly as you examine to allow you to see into the angle more clearly. Avoid excessive pressure as this will artificially open an angle if using a four mirror lens (indentation gonioscopy – see below) or falsely narrow an angle with the bigger Goldmann by pressing on the sclera at the limbus. If you are struggling to see the angle ask the patient to look slightly into the direction of the mirror you are using, as this slight movement can help you to see over the top of the iris and see right into the area of interest.

One of the benefits of the four-mirror lenses such as the Zeiss is that because they have a surface contact area of less than the total corneal surface you can use them for indentation gonioscopy. Axial pressure on the central cornea with the lens will flatten it and force aqueous into the angle (Fig. 6.5). This will open the angle and hopefully allow you to visualize the TM. Sometimes prolonged angle closure will result in apposition of the iris tissue to the angle or posterior cornea and adhesions will develop (peripheral anterior synechiae).

It will take practice – be patient.

The first key question you need to ask yourself is whether you can see the TM for 360°. If you can, then the angle is open. If you cannot, then the amount of TM which is obscured by either the anatomy of the peripheral iris (primary angle closure (PAC)) or by pathological processes such as synechiae (secondary angle closure), will dictate the patient's clinical course. There is no definitive guidance as to what is an 'occludable' angle, i.e. which angles can predispose

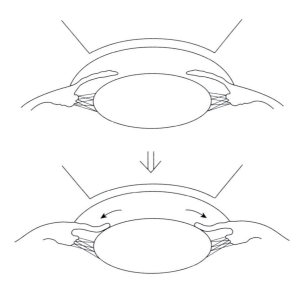

Figure 6.5 Diagram showing the principle of indentation gonioscopy. Because the lens surface is of a smaller diameter than the cornea, pressure upon it can displace aqueous into the angle thereby opening it and revealing the angle anatomy.

or turn into PAC. There is some consensus that if less than 90° of TM is visible then there is the *potential* that PAC may occur (see Chapter 22).

Grading the angle

You need to now grade the angle and so you or other clinicians can document changes if they occur. There are numerous different systems; the simplest is the Shaffer staging. The easiest way to do this is to concentrate on the most posterior structure you can see. The angle is usually documented for all four quadrants. If you can see the ciliary body it is a grade 4 – wide open (Fig. 6.6). If you can see the scleral spur but no ciliary body it is a grade 3. Visible TM makes it a grade 2 while if no trabecular meshwork is visible but you can see Schwalbe's line the grade is 1. When no structures are visible at all the grade is zero and the angle is effectively closed. Grades 1 and 0 are occludable angles. Remember that the superior angle is normally the narrowest.

If you cannot see the TM, ie. grade is narrower than 2, *decide why*. Possible causes include:

- Iridocorneal angle anatomy. In this situation the iridocorneal angle is physiologically narrow, i.e. the angle between peripheral iris and inner surface of cornea is narrow due to all or a combination of: the shape of the anterior chamber; the short axial length; the flat cornea; and a large lens. The key is whether this can turn into a pathological narrowing, i.e. PAC. Sometimes the angle can open on indentation gonioscopy excluding the presence of PAS. This has important clinical implications as if the angle is not completely stuck down (due to synechiae) laser iridotomy may open it. Cataract surgery in this situation may also have a role to play, as removing the lens will inevitably open such angles (see Chapter 22).

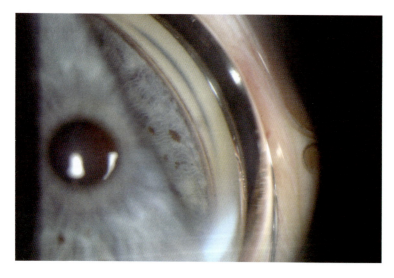

Figure 6.6 Open angle – grade 4 on gonioscopy. The scleral spur is clearly seen as the bright white band. This makes the structure posterior to it the ciliary body and the area just anterior to it the pigmented trabecular meshwork. Schwalbe's line is not clearly seen due to its lack of pigment.

- Peripheral anterior synechiae (PAS). These are pathological adhesions between the peripheral iris and the angle structures or the endothelium of the far peripheral cornea. It is easy to confuse iris processes for PAS. Iris processes are normal strands of iris tissue that extend from the iris surface into the TM. They tend to be quite thin and discrete. Although they may be numerous they do not usually form broad bands and you can see the underlying structures between them. PAS are wide bands of iris tissue and tend to obscure angle anatomy (Fig. 6.7). PAS can occur after recurrent intraocular inflammation, or after prolonged narrowing of the angle with tissue apposition. Inferior PAS are seen in patients with chronic or recurrent iritis probably because gravity and aqueous currents cause inflammatory cells and protein-aceous matter to settle inferiorly. PAS can also form in association with neovascularization.
- Angle neovascularization. You will often see normal blood vessels at gonioscopy – the key is to differentiate these from pathology. As a general rule, 'normal' blood vessels never cross the scleral spur. They are usually radial, running through the superficial iris stroma, with few branches, and are seen more often in patients with light-colored irides. New angle vessels occur due to ischemic processes resulting in release of vasoproliferative factors stimulating growth of fibrovascular tissue in the iridocorneal angle. This process usually occurs second-ary to ischemic retinopathies such as diabetic retinopathy, secondary to a central retinal vein occlusion or as a result of an ocular ischemic syndrome. The new vessels sprout from the normal vasculature of the iris and the CB. They are fine, and follow an irregular branching course, beginning as fine lacy fronds (Fig. 6.8). They have a predeliction for areas of high aqueous flow (as the aqueous carries the vasoproliferative factors) and thus occur first at the pupil margin and then on the iris surface and in the angle. Unlike the case in disc neovascu-larization, bleeding is not the major concern with angle vessels. Accompanying the new vessels is a fibrous membrane which acts as a scaffold for their growth. This is initially clear and extends across the angle blocking aqueous outflow, resulting in an apparently open angle but raised IOP. As this fibrovascular membrane grows and becomes more substantial, contraction occurs and the angle closes (synechial angle closure) obscuring view of the TM and totally blocking aqueous outflow. Judicious and rapid treatment of the ischemic process can reverse the neovascularization, causing this membrane to fade away restoring patency of the angle. This will only be possible in the early stages of the angle pathology and highlights again the need for accurate and thorough gonioscopy in at-risk cases.

Other considerations

Once you've had a good look at all four quadrants and graded the angle you need to move on to look for other clues as to the presence of pathology.

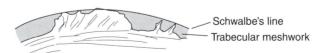

Figure 6.7 Diagram showing the appearance of peripheral anterior synechiae on gonioscopy. Here areas of trabecular meshwork are visible; with further synechiae formation, however, the trabecular meshwork can be completely obscured and the angle can close fully.

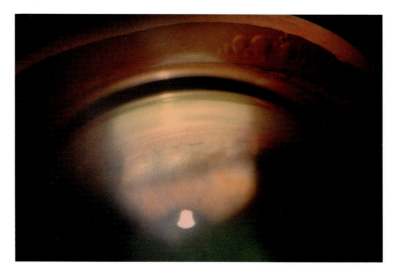

Figure 6.8 Neovascularization on gonioscopy. Color photograph of gonioscopic view showing fine branching neovascularization of the angle.

The iris

The iris contour in the normal eye is slightly convex due to it following the shape of the lens. The iris makes contact with the lens surface at the pupil and aqueous has to overcome this contact to move into the anterior chamber. This creates a pressure difference between the front and back of the iris with more pressure required posteriorly to push the iris out of the way at the pupil and allow normal aqueous flow from back to front. This pressure difference causes the iris to bow forward and results in a physiological element of pupil block which occurs in all normal eyes (Fig. 6.9). If there is a peripheral gap in the iris (for example due to an iridotomy) then the pressure difference disappears and this bowing does not occur. In aphakia or pseudophakia the iris–lens contact is abolished and no pressure differential occurs resulting in a flat iris contour. Hypermetropic eyes tend to have crowded anterior structures with shallower ACs, narrower angles and more pronounced iris convexity. In myopes the AC tends to be deeper with more posterior positioning of the lens–iris diaphragm. This gives the iris a flat contour as it runs from the angle direct to the pupil margin. Indeed, because there is space behind the iris it can sometimes bow backwards giving a concave appearance. The iris is often seen to insert quite far back giving a nice view of the ciliary body all the way round. These are great cases to practice your gonioscopy on and get an understanding of the structures you are looking for.

Plateau iris configuration is typified by an iris root that inserts just behind the scleral spur. This is not a problem as such an insertion behind the TM usually means an open angle. From the insertion, however, the peripheral iris angulates sharply anteriorly, creating a relatively narrow iridocorneal angle. Once it reaches the peak it turns and heads towards the pupil margin with a flat contour (the plateau). This is not an easy diagnosis to make and it is more important

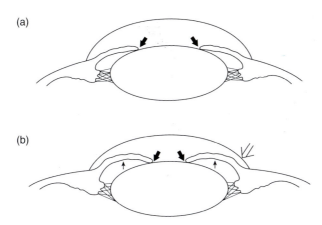

(a)

(b)

Figure 6.9 Diagram of pupil block. (a) The normal physiological situation. There is a certain degree of 'normal' pupil block which occurs where the iris sits in contact with the lens surface (solid arrows). This is overcome by normal flow dynamics and the aqueous enters the anterior chamber and drains into the angle. (b) Pupil block. The pupil margin now blocks flow of aqueous into the anterior chamber (solid arrows) and the aqueous collects in the posterior chamber pushing the iris forward (line arrows). The angle subsequently closes (open arrow) and angle closure occurs with raised IOP.

to identify the narrow, potentially occludable angle. The only way to definitively make the diagnosis is to undertake prophylactic iridotomy and then find that the patient still develops PAC. Although the morphology can give a clue, the diagnosis tends to be based on clinical course in most patients. The use of ultrasound biomicroscopy technology may help us make this morphological diagnosis with more confidence (see Chapter 22).

Angle pigmentation

The amount of pigmentation in the angle should be documented and graded 0 to 4. There is usually more pigment inferiorly than superiorly due to the relative increased function of the lower TM, and its density tends to increase with age. Pigmentation is browny/black and finely granular. The pigment tends to concentrate on the posterior two thirds of the TM (hence the name pigmented TM). Some angles are so depigmented that it makes determination of the anatomical structures extremely difficult. In elderly patients, PXF is the most common cause of excessive trabecular pigmentation, especially if the pigmentation is asymmetrical between the eyes. In younger persons with more bilaterally symmetric trabecular hyperpigmentation, PDS is the most likely cause. Previous trauma and intraocular surgery can result in excessive pigmentation. Very rarely tumors of the iris or ciliary body can result in such changes. If there is a great degree of (usually pathological) pigmentation it can spread anteriorly beyond the TM resulting in deposition of pigment at or just anterior to Schwalbe's line. This can form a discrete line called Sampaolesi's line (Fig. 6.10).

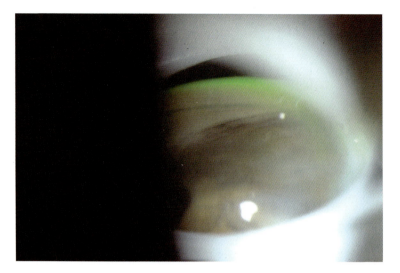

Figure 6.10 Sampaolesi's line on gonioscopy. An excessively pigmented angle with localized deposition of pigment just anterior to Schwalbe's line. The angle is open with clearly visualized trabecular meshwork.

Angle recession

One other angle abnormality of which to be aware is angle recession. This occurs from traumatic separation of the longitudinal muscles from the circular muscles of the CB. Angle recession may be localized or involve the entire 360° of the angle. It can be hard to identify if the amount of recession is uniform as the angle can simply look wide open. Compare quadrants within the eye and between the two eyes to detect pathological differences. Look carefully for other signs of previous trauma and ask the patient! Angle recession is a risk factor for elevated IOP at any time after the event. The more angle recession the greater the risk of developing raised IOP in the future but it is far from certain that this will occur even if the entire angle is recessed.

Cyclodialysis cleft

Blunt trauma may result in a tear causing separation of the ciliary body from the scleral spur. This is called cyclodialysis and results in low-resistance drainage of aqueous into the supra-choroidal space causing a low IOP and hypotony with potential visual loss.

Look carefully for a localized increase in the width of the scleral spur. This apparent widening occurs because the ciliary body has been ripped from the underlying surface and you are seeing sclera in the defect. In a soft eye this can be very difficult to see. The only way to be sure (and undertake a proper examination in such situations) is to take the patient to theater and form the AC with an ophthalmic viscoelastic and use gonioscopy under the operating microscope.

References

1. Van Herrick W, Shaffer RN, Schwartz A. Estimation of width of angle of anterior chamber. Am J Ophthalmol 1969; 68: 626–629.
2. Kashiwagi K, Tokunaga T, Iwase A, Yamamoto T, Tsukahara S. Agreement between peripheral anterior chamber depth evaluation using the van Herrick technique and angle width evaluation using the Shaffer system in Japanese. Jpn J Ophthalmol 2005; 49: 134–136.

Chapter 7

Evaluation of the optic nerve head

Why should I read this chapter?

Optic nerve assessment is key to the diagnosis of glaucoma. When considering the triad of glaucoma – raised IOP, visual-field loss and optic disc changes – the optic disc changes are arguably the most important. You can have a normal IOP but still have glaucoma (normal-tension glaucoma) and you can have a normal visual field but still have glaucoma (preperimetric glaucoma). You can also have abnormal visual fields due to other causes *but* you cannot have a normal disc and still have glaucoma. It is of course this definite detection of a 'normal' disc which causes the diagnostic difficulty.

Detailed and thorough examination of the optic nerve head is paramount in the management of glaucoma.

IMPORTANT: Imaging techniques do not take the place of clinical examination.

You cannot rely on photographs or machines to assess an optic nerve in isolation. Any such devices are adjuncts to your care and may be helpful in documenting and quantifying changes or progression. The clinician must be highly competent at assessing the optic nerve to:

(1) Distinguish normal from abnormal
(2) Make a diagnosis of glaucoma
(3) Detect clinical signs of potential glaucoma progression

In the presence of a visual-field defect any changes in the disc should correspond in anatomical location and severity to account for the perimetric loss. If the discrepancies do not match up, the clinician should question whether the visual-field defect is true or artifactual. Then look for any other pathology that may be causing it. In particular clinicians should be always on the look out for post-chiasmal causes of a visual-field loss, for example brain tumors.

Normal anatomy

Retinal ganglion cell axons make up almost all of the neuroretinal rim (NRR) tissue of the optic disc. These axons sweep in from all parts of the retina travelling in the retinal nerve fiber layer (RNFL). At the optic disc they are required to shift from the retinal plane by 90° to enter the optic nerve as it heads back towards the brain. A fine complex of capillaries surround and infiltrate the optic disc to provide oxygen and nutrition to the axons as they traverse this area.

This blood supply and the axoplasm within the axons give the NRR an orange–red appearance. Glial cells and astrocytes provide connective tissue support to these axons. Inevitably when the ganglion cell fibers turn to enter the nerve they leave a dip in the centre. This is called the optic cup and is usually devoid of tissue. The color of the NRR is partly due to the fact that you are effectively looking at the barrels of the axons that form the optic nerve. Within the central cup there are no such axons and you are visualizing the lamina cribrosa more clearly. The lamina cribrosa is the sieve-like area of the scleral shell which allows the exit of the nerve fibers which form the optic nerve. It is white and thus the cup usually appears paler than the surrounding NRR.

Evaluation techniques

True evaluation of the optic nerve requires dilated fundus examination with stereopsis. Monocular techniques, such as the direct ophthalmoscope, rely on clues as to the position and size of the neuroretinal rim. Without a three-dimensional view, the examiner relies on two-dimensional clues, such color changes between the NRR and the cup and the course of the blood vessels as they travel over the edge of the disc rim, to gauge the position and size of the cup and the health of the rim. Monocular examination techniques are sub-optimal and can result in underestimation of the true degree of glaucoma damage. The only real benefit of the direct ophthalmoscope is the degree of magnification it offers allowing a close-up view of the NRR. It is an important skill to have, however, as there are some glaucoma patients who cannot sit at the slit lamp and their glaucoma management will rely on this technique.

Stereoscopic methods allow the examiner to get a detailed impression of the topographic contour of the whole optic disc with accurate evaluation of the optic cup and NRR tissue.

The ideal examination technique is via the use of the slit lamp biomicroscope with a non-contact condensing lens. 90 D, 78 D and 60 D lenses are available for use. Again this technique requires practice and the examiner has to remember that the image obtained is inverted and reversed. The superior part of the disc when visualized is actually the inferior disc and vice versa. At this stage it is important to once more emphasize the fact that the initial glaucoma assessment is a full ophthalmic evaluation. The clinician has also to examine the macula and the peripheral retina to look for concurrent ocular morbidity. Any concurrent macular pathology can have significant implications in the management of the glaucoma patient. Visual loss attributable to a macular cause can affect the patient's ability to do visual-field tests (Fig. 7.1). A peripheral retinopathy or retinal scar can be the sole cause of a visual-field defect (Fig. 7.2). A myopic patient who may or may not have glaucoma may have a staphyloma (Fig. 7.3) or even a giant retinal tear which is a direct short-term threat to their vision. It is important that the retinal peripheries are examined at outset in every new patient. Naturally future changes in the patient's condition may necessitate further formal dilated examination of the posterior pole and the peripheral retina.

The 78 D and 60 D lenses provide good magnification and allow close up optimal viewing of the ONH. The 90 D provides a wider view and may be useful when assessing the RNFL as it allows a broader picture and may facilitate detection of areas of NFL loss. In general the 78 D probably gives the best view of the ONH for glaucoma examination.

Various contact lenses may also be used to examine the ONH. These are more invasive techniques requiring coupling agents and thus tend to be less user and patient friendly. The only benefit is that the image obtained is not inverted.

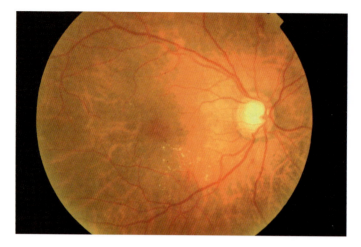

Figure 7.1 Concurrent morbidity. Color fundus photograph showing a resolving inferior macular branch retinal vein occlusion in an eye with glaucoma. Such comorbidity may be missed unless dilated fundus examination is carried out and may even be the cause of sudden worsening of the visual-field defect.

It is important that the examination of the ONH is methodical and systematic at each visit. If assessing a follow-up then try and avoid biasing yourself by looking at the previous medical notes. Make your own decisions regarding the state of the ONH and only then compare this to previous examinations.

Of course there are some discs, such as highly myopic discs, which are virtually impossible to assess (Fig. 7.4).

Potential findings

The presence of a cup in the optic disc is not in itself pathological. Even high degrees of optic disc cupping may be physiological, i.e. normal for that patient. Previously, simply documenting the vertical cup-to-disc ratio (vCDR) (the vertical dimensions of the cup compared with the vertical dimensions of the disc producing a ratio) was adequate for optic disc assessment. As glaucoma worsens the cup-to-disc ratio increases.

Cup-to-disc ratios (CDR)

The CDR is a useful and widely used measure of glaucomatous changes in the optic nerve head. This ratio compares the vertical size of the cup to the overall top to bottom size of the optic disc (Fig. 7.5). Normal or physiological cups are extremely common and the differentiation between pathological and physiological cupping is a vital skill in the armamentarium of the glaucoma clinician. As a general rule the greater the CDR the greater the likelihood of glaucoma. However, *and it is an enormous 'however'*, the CDR is highly variable and dependent upon the

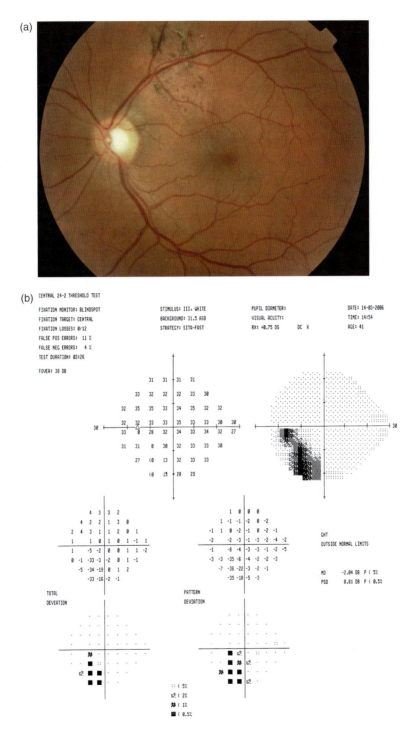

Figure 7.2 Scar causing visual-field defect. (a) Color fundus photograph showing a superior pigmentary retinal scar. (b) 24-2 Humphreys visual field delineating a corresponding visual-field defect.

(a)

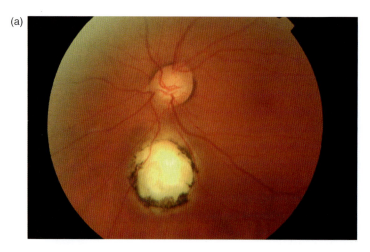

(b)

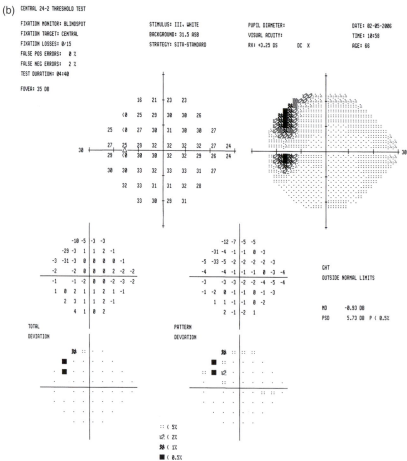

Figure 7.3 Staphyloma causing visual-field defect. (a) Color fundus photograph showing an inferior staphyloma in a myopic patient. Note that the optic disc is physiologically cupped. (b) 24-2 Humphreys visual field revealing a corresponding visual-field defect.

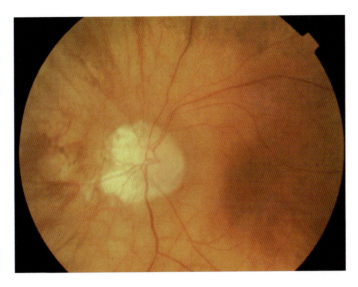

Figure 7.4 Uninterpretable disc. Color fundus photograph showing a highly myopic disc with extensive peripapillary atrophy. Such discs are almost impossible to assess accurately.

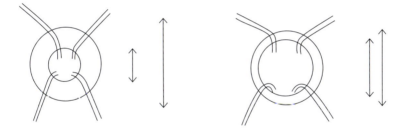

Figure 7.5 Diagram of cup-to-disc ratios. The CDR is described according to the vertical dimensions of the cup itself compared to the overall vertical size of the disc. The CDRs here are 0.5 and 0.8 respectively.

size of the optic disc and the number of nerve fibers which enter the disc and turn to exit the eye as the optic nerve.

Concentrating on the vertical dimension only can be problematic. The whole NRR should be assessed at each visit as, although the whole vertical cup dimensions may be static, the patient could be developing widening of their horizontal cup or thinning and notching of the NRR in the oblique axis. Look at the whole rim carefully and document any areas of thinning. Consider documenting the CDR for the axis corresponding to the thinnest part of the NRR.

It is now clearly recognized that this simple observation of vCDR is flawed and used in isolation is of limited use. Larger optic discs can carry the same number of nerve fibers as smaller discs. Thus when the same number of nerve fibers turn the corner and enter the optic nerve they may fill the smaller disc (resulting in no cup) while simply lining the edges of the larger cup (resulting in a space/cup centrally). Large optic discs may thus have significant physiological cups with no loss of retinal nerve fiber numbers.[1] They are effectively normal discs with the

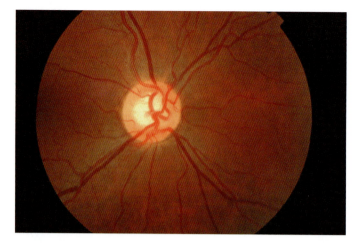

Figure 7.6 Physiological cup. Color photograph of a physiological cup. The ISNT rule is obeyed, the disc is large and the neuroretinal rim is thick and intact throughout the circumference of the disc.

appearance of glaucomatous cupping. As a very general rule, the larger the disc the larger the 'allowed' cup.

In a suspected physiological cup, thorough assessment of the NRR should reveal no evidence of focal loss or notching, the ISNT rule should be obeyed (see below) and there should be no sign of any RNFL defect (Fig. 7.6). The other eye should show a similar disc and cup appearance unless the disc in that eye is of a different size.

Measurement of the size of the disc is thus an important parameter and it should be taken into account whenever considering the CDR or the observed width of the NRR.[2,3]

Measuring disc size

There is considerable variation in the physiologic disc size in the normal population.[4] Black people tend to have larger optic discs and larger optic cups than white people.[5] The optic disc is also 2–3% larger in men than in women.[6] Large discs may have large cups[5,6] with a greater CDR and slightly more nerve fibers.[7] The reverse is true for small discs, which normally have smaller cups and fewer nerve fibers.

One simple method to give a rough indication of disc size is to use arterial blood vessel width as a comparator. The clinician can estimate the number of arterial blood vessel widths that can fit across the horizontal dimension of the optic disc. In a normal-sized disc, this is approximately 10–12. As a rough guide a small disc will have 10 or less and a large disc will have in excess of 12.

A more accurate and reproducible technique involves projecting a thin slit from the slit lamp and measuring the vertical dimension of the disc as the slit overlies it. Dilate the patient to allow a good view and adequate stereopsis. The slit is narrowed and brightened. The beam is aligned axially and a 78 D lens is used to project the slit into the eye under visualization. The beam is moved to overlie the disc and is progressively reduced in length until the top and bottom of the

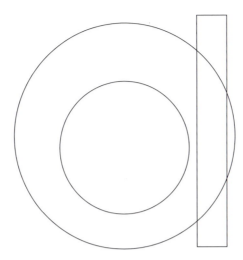

Figure 7.7 Diagram showing a disc being measured. The slit lamp beam is shortened until it just spans the vertical disc distance and then a reading is taken. The size measured will be dependent on the type of lens utilized.

Table 7.1 Correction factors for common lenses.

Lens name	Image magnification factor
Volk 60D Lens	×1.15
Volk 78D Lens	×0.93
Volk 90D Lens	×0.76

beam precisely fit the vertical dimensions of the disc (Fig. 7.7). Sometimes the slit can 'disappear' into the nerve making precise measurement difficult. It is helpful to move the slit to the side of the nerve intermittently to see whether you are correctly measuring the full height of the disc. Once the examiner is happy with the slit height the measurement is read off the slit lamp in millimeters. This does not translate directly into true disc size as it will need to be multiplied by a corrective factor dependent upon the type of lens utilized. Different lenses have different magnification and this must be factored in to your size assessment (Table 7.1).

A moderate sized cup and thus an intermediate CDR in a large disc may be normal while the same sized cup and CDR in a very small disc may be highly pathological (Fig. 7.8).

Again it is worth emphasis that you must not simply focus on the vertical CDR in isolation. You are only looking at the top and bottom sections of optic disc and NRR when you use the CDR tool. You have to methodically assess the whole rim so as not to miss a focal lesion or progression of a previously noted abnormal area in another part of the NRR. Watch out particularly for notches or aquired optic disc pits (Fig. 7.9), adherence to the ISNT rule (see below), optic disc hemorrhages, or focal pallor.

In addition to these NRR features the clinician should assess for asymmetry in optic nerve cupping between the two eyes, for the presence of diffuse pallor, for the presence of RNFL defects, and for the presence and type of peripapillary atrophy (PPA).

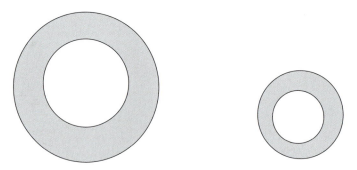

Figure 7.8 A moderate-sized cup and thus an intermediate CDR in a large disc may be normal while the same sized cup and CDR in a very small disc may be highly pathological. Two discs are shown. Both have a CDR of 0.6. The larger disc is probably physiologically cupped, however this degree of cupping in a much smaller disc may be glaucomatous. Note the difference in neuroretinal rim area between the two discs despite identical CDRs. Unless measured, this difference in disc size may be missed.

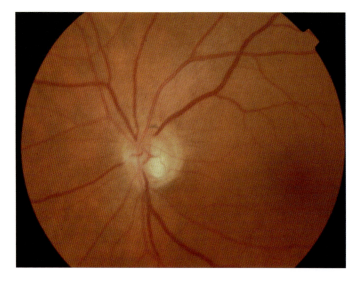

Figure 7.9 Optic disc pit. An acquired inferior optic disc pit. The vessels are seen to dip into this area and then reappear centrally.

ISNT rule

Using this tool is a useful clinical exercise in deciding whether a disc is glaucomatous.[8] Normal discs have a thicker inferior NRR when compared to the superior NRR. In turn the superior NRR is thicker than the nasal NRR which is thicker than the temporal NRR. Hence the ISNT rule represents the normal relationship between the thickest part of the NRR progressing to the thinnest part:

I (inf) S (sup) N (nasal) T (temporal) NRR.

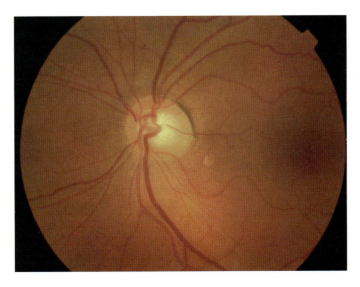

Figure 7.10 ISNT rule not obeyed. Color fundus photograph of an optic disc which does not obey the ISNT rule. The superior rim is thicker than the inferior rim.

This simply represents the anatomical arrangement of the eye and the volume of nerve fibers projecting from the relative portions of the retina. The inferior retina is the largest area and thus supplies the NRR with the greatest complement of nerve fibers. The superior retina is the next greatest area, then the nasal and finally the temporal retina. The temporal part of the disc receives mostly nerve fibers coming horizontally across from the nasal macula. The majority of the nerve fibers from the temporal retina arc around the macula and join the superior or inferior portions of the NRR. If the superior rim is thinner than the inferior rim a suspicion of glaucoma should be raised (Fig. 7.10).

Notches of the neuroretinal rim

Generalized concentric enlargement of the cup is the most common optic disc change in progressive glaucoma (Fig. 7.11).[9] Notching is seen most frequently in the inferior NRR[10,11] and refers to localized thinning of a portion of the NRR which outpaces generalized rim loss. Such inferior notches are usually associated with superior well localized scotoma (Fig. 7.12). Rim is often first lost at the superior or inferior poles resulting in vertical cup enlargement. This may be due to the fact that histopathologically there is less supportive connective tissue at the superior and inferior portions of the disc resulting in reduced mechanical support for the nerve fibers in those regions.[12,13] Sectoral loss of NRR may be highly localized involving one clock hour or more diffuse involving several clock hours but relatively sparing other parts of the rim (Fig. 7.13).

Concentrate carefully on the superotemporal and inferotemporal portions of the disc as this is where the glaucoma damage is usually most evident. These portions of damage correspond to the inferior and superior arcuate glaucomatous visual-field defects respectively.

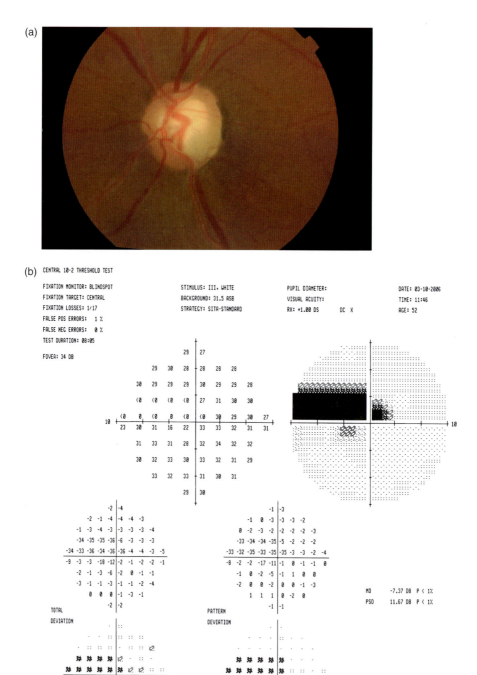

Figure 7.11 Disc notch. (a) Color fundus photograph of the optic nerve showing a distinct notch in the inferior neuro-retinal rim. (b) 10-2 Humphreys visual field showing a localized superior scotoma fitting with the position of the optic disc notch.

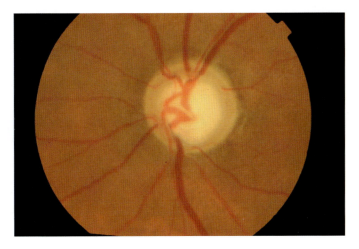

Figure 7.12 Diffuse loss of neuroretinal rim. This glaucomatous disc demonstrates diffuse loss of the NRR and a markedly enlarged CDR.

Generally speaking, the smaller the NRR area, the greater the likelihood of glaucomatous optic neuropathy. Of course it is vital to factor in the size of the optic nerve head when considering rim area. If NRR area was a constant across all patients then the determination of glaucoma would be easier. Unfortunately it is known that larger discs have a greater NRR area than their smaller counterparts due to a greater number of nerve fibers. Paradoxically the NRR area may appear clinically depleted in larger discs due to the distribution of this larger volume of NRR over the greater circumferential area.

Asymmetry of disc cupping

In normals, the CDR is usually symmetrical between the two eyes of an individual[14,15] with 99% of the normal population having a less than 0.2 difference between the CDRs of each eye.[14] CDR asymmetry is a key hallmark of glaucoma.[16] Assuming that the disc sizes are the same (and assuming that you have diligently measured them) then the discs should have approximately the same size cup. Naturally if one of the discs is significantly larger than the other then this may be the sole factor accounting for the difference in CDR between the two eyes.

Optic disc pallor

Glaucoma is an optic neuropathy with the end result being optic atrophy. This atrophy is inevitably accompanied by pallor. Pallor occurs because of a selective loss of the non-collagenous connective, neural and vascular tissue in the ONH. This allows more of the collagenous component to show through resulting in relative whiteness or pallor. As a general rule

(a)

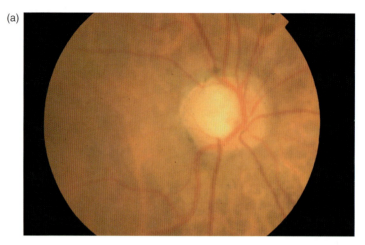

(b)

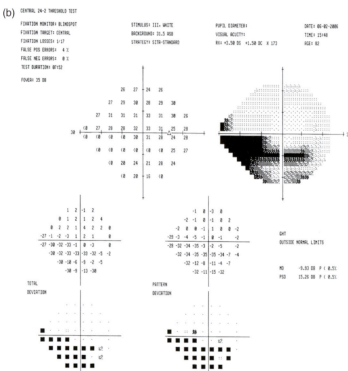

Figure 7.13 Broad neuroretinal rim loss. (a) Color fundus photograph of the optic disc showing broad superior loss of the NRR but relative sparing of the rest of the rim. (b) 24–2 Humphreys visual field showing a corresponding inferior scotoma.

in glaucoma the area of pallor is less than the area of cupping. It is important to avoid concentrating purely on the area of central pallor as the examiner may miss the larger extent of cupping.

The remaining NRR, even in reasonably advanced glaucoma, retains a degree of pinkness. Watch out for NRR pallor or an optic disc which is diffusely pale. It can sometimes be difficult to determine the true color of the disc due to lens opacities. Conversely in pseudophakic patients the disc may look pale simply due to the fact that the IOL is optically clear (Fig. 7.14). It is often helpful to compare the color carefully with the other eye, however this relies on the assumption that the other disc is not equally pale.

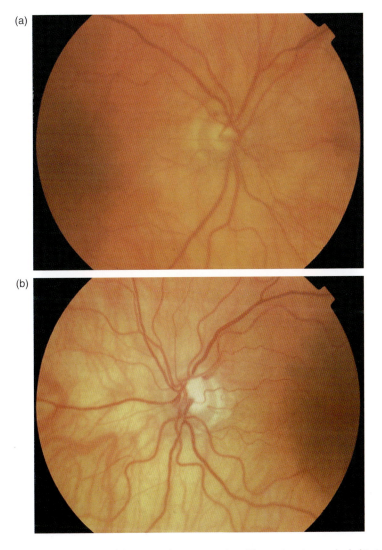

(a)

(b)

Figure 7.14 (a) & (b) Right and left eyes of the same glaucoma patient. The patient is pseudophakic in the left eye and has a cataract in the right eye. The color difference in optic nerves is clear but it is unknown whether this apparent disc pallor on the left is due solely to the pseudophakic status.

Disc hemorrhages

ODHs are not only found in glaucoma patients. A recent large-scale study from Japan found a prevalence of 0.2% in non-glaucoma patients versus an 8.2% prevalence in established glaucoma.[17] The exact pathophysiology of ODHs is surprisingly unknown. Their occurrence may be related to microinfarcts of the peripapillary NFL with a subsequent reperfusion injury resulting in rupture of a compromised capillary. They have been found to occur more frequently in diabetics or patients taking aspirin,[18] however, this may simply represent the greater time to resolution of these hemorrhages and thus the greater likelihood of picking them up. Without doubt these hemorrhages come and go, resolving after approximately 6 weeks. Disc hemorrhages appear to be related to glaucoma progression, particularly in patients with NTG.[19–21] In addition the visual field loss occurs in the area corresponding to the location of the ODH usually with some degree of lag between the onset of the disc hemorrhage and the progression of the visual field.[19] Curiously ODHs seem to occur more frequently in glaucoma eyes with a lower IOP than those with a higher IOP.[18]

These hemorrhages occur most frequently at the inferior pole of the disc, followed by the superior then temporal poles. They are usually located on the optic disc or in the immediate peripapillary area and tend to be flame shaped when within the retinal nerve fiber layer and more blot-like on the disc itself (Fig. 7.15). Occasionally resolving hemorrhages may be visible as tiny splinter hemorrhages. The detection of ODHs is enhanced by pupil dilatation and thus they may frequently be missed at routine follow-ups.

A disc hemorrhage in a patient who is a glaucoma suspect should prompt initiation of treatment. A patient with established glaucoma who develops a disc hemorrhage should have their level of glaucoma control seriously readdressed with consideration to lowering IOP further.

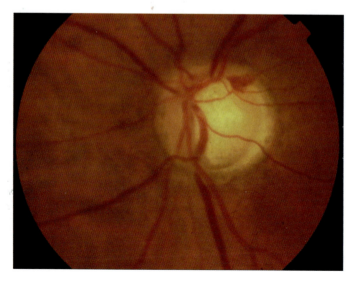

Figure 7.15 Optic disc hemorrhage. A glaucomatous optic disc with a large superior ODH overlying the neuroretinal rim.

Naturally should this require surgery then it may be more prudent to await any evidence of subsequent visual-field loss before embarking on and accepting the risks of surgery.

Peripapillary atrophy

A scleral lip commonly surrounds the optic nerve head and is seen as a thin regular circumferential band of white. It represents the anterior extension of the sclera lying between the choroid and nerve head. The next area, if present, is usually a crescent of depigmentation caused by retraction of the RPE layer next to the disc allowing relative baring of the sclera. This is called beta-zone peripapillary atrophy (PPA) and is a common finding in glaucomatous eyes (Fig. 7.16). There is some evidence to suggest that beta-zone PPA may be a risk factor for glaucoma damage.

Theoretically, the absence of a fully formed outer blood–retinal barrier in the area of bared sclera may allow vasoactive agents access to the ONH capillaries affecting autoregulation and causing or exacerbating any glaucomatous nerve head vascular abnormalities. Alpha-zone PPA is seen as a crescent of increased pigmentation and has less clinical significance in the setting of glaucoma (Fig. 7.17).

The presence and the size of PPA may relate to the development of subsequent optic disc or visual-field damage in patients with OHT[22,23], and furthermore progression of this PPA may be the first sign of glaucoma in OHT patients.[24] There is evidence that progression of PPA is associated with progressive optic disc damage and worsening visual-field loss in glaucoma, potentially making it a marker for progression.[25]

The area of NRR adjacent to the PPA is at particular risk of damage[26] and this area should undergo rigorous scrutiny by the clinician.

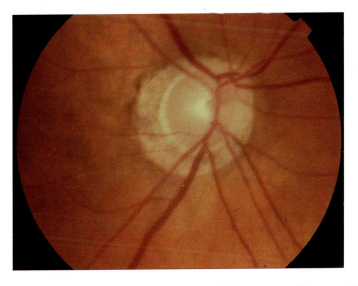

Figure 7.16 Beta-zone peripapillary atrophy. Color fundus photograph showing typical beta-zone PPA around the optic nerve head.

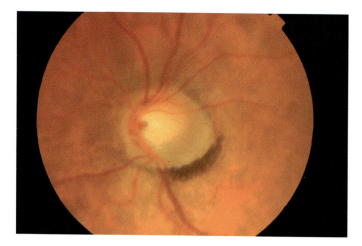

Figure 7.17 Alpha-zone peripapillary atrophy. Disc photograph showing a crescent of pigmentation characteristic of alpha-zone PPA.

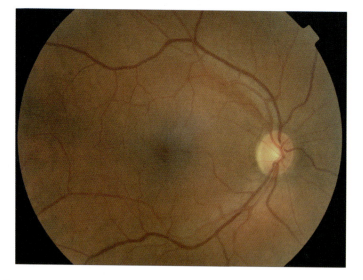

Figure 7.18 Nerve fiber layer defect. Color fundus photograph of a patient's right eye. A RNFL wedge defect is clearly seen arching out from the superior portion of the optic disc.

Retinal nerve fiber layer

The assessment of the RNFL can be very useful in separating those eyes that are normal from those with early glaucomatous optic nerve changes.[27–29]

Loss of nerve fibers which leads to thinning of the NRR may first manifest as a visible defect in the RNFL. These appear as dark stripes or wedge-shaped defects in the usual uniformly reflective sheen of the RNFL. These dark patches usually follow the normal retinal striations and are best seen at the transition point between normal and abnormal areas, i.e. light and dark (Fig. 7.18). Focal defects may be seen in association with ODHs[30,31], and correlate highly with

NRR loss[32] and with visual-field defects in glaucoma.[33,34] Diffuse defects are harder to visualize than focal defects as the generalized loss of sheen/RNFL may be hard to detect. Comparing the superior and inferior peripapillary RNFL or the two eyes may be helpful in improving pick-up rate of diffuse loss.

Examination of the RNFL is best carried out using slit lamp biomicroscopy with red-free (green) illumination. It is important to wash out residual fluorescein from the tear film as this can reduce contrast detection and moreover the red-free light may cause some degree of fluorescence that will affect your view. The RNFL immediately around the disc is the area of interest as it is the thickest and thus any focal or diffuse loss will be most obvious in this region.

Focus on the retinal striations. Look carefully for wedge-shaped defects and diffuse loss among the characteristic curvilinear striations of the nerve fibers. Wedge-shaped defects will be detected due to the sharp transition to normal RNFL at the edge of the defect.

Nerve fiber layer loss is a useful tool in younger patients. As individuals age they lose more and more nerve fibers as part of normal aging and thus the detection of diffuse loss has limited clinical significance unless supported by other clinical findings or marked asymmetry between eyes.

Both diffuse loss and wedge-shaped defects may occur years before visual field deterioration, emphasizing the need to detect these pathological changes early. The presence of a RNFL defect in a glaucoma suspect or OHT patient should increase the index of suspicion for glaucoma and lower the threshold for treatment.

Conclusion

There is wide variability of optic disc appearance in the normal population resulting in much overlap between a glaucomatous and normal ONH, particularly in early glaucoma. One feature of an ONH is not enough to make a diagnosis of glaucoma and thus all the clinical information available needs to be taken into account before management decisions are made. The clinician needs to consider the IOP, the visual fields, the gonioscopic appearance and numerous patient characteristics before embarking on a treatment regimen or altering a pre-existing one.

There are many imaging devices available which aim to assess morphology and give the user information as to the normality of the optic disc or nerve fiber layer. *These do not replace clinical examination.* There are many problems associated with such devices and interpretation of the evidence they present may lead to significant errors of judgment. Remember you are treating the patient and not their print-outs. Clinical examination is essential and no amount of clever technology will replace a thorough, methodical and systematic assessment of the disc.

References

1. Crowston JG, Hopley CR, Healey PR, Lee A, Mitchell P. The effect of optic disc diameter on vertical cup to disc ratio percentiles in a population based cohort: the Blue Mountains Eye Study. Br J Ophthalmol 2004; 88: 766–770.

2. Garway-Heath DF, Ruben ST, Viswanathan A, Hitchings RA. Vertical cup/disc ratio in relation to optic disc size: its value in the assessment of the glaucoma suspect. Br J Ophthalmol 1998; 82: 1118–1124.

3. Healey PR, Mitchell P, Smith W, Wang JJ. Relationship between cup-disc ratio and optic disc diameter: the Blue Mountains Eye Study. Aust N Z J Ophthalmol. 1997; 25: S99–101.

4. Jonas JB, Gusek GC, Guggenmoos-Holzmann I, Naumann GO. Variability of the real dimensions of normal human optic discs. Graefe's Arch Clin Exp Ophthalmol 1988; 226: 332–336.

5. Quigley HA, Brown AE, Morrison JD, Drance SM. The size and shape of the optic disc in normal human eyes. Arch Ophthalmol 1990; 108: 51–57.

6. Varma R, Tielsch JM, Quigley HA, et al. Race-, age-, gender-, and refractive error-related differences in the normal optic disc. Arch Ophthalmol 1994; 112: 1068–1076.

7. Hancox MD. Optic disc size, an important consideration in the glaucoma evaluation. Clin Eye Vis Care 1999; 1: 59–62.

8. Harizman N, Oliveira C, Chiang A, et al. The ISNT rule and differentiation of normal from glaucomatous eyes. Arch Ophthalmol 2006; 124: 1579–1583.

9. Pederson JE, Anderson DR. The mode of progressive disc cupping in ocular hypertensive and glaucoma. Arch Ophthalmol 1980; 98: 490.

10. Airaksinen PJ, Drance SM, Schulzer M. Neuroretinal rim areas in early glaucoma. Am J Ophthalmol 1985; 99: 1.

11. Spaeth G, Hitchings RA, Sivalingam E. The optic disc in glaucoma: pathogenetic correlation of five patterns of cupping in chronic open-angle glaucoma. Symposium on Glaucoma. Trans Am Acad Ophthalmol Otolaryngol 1976; 81: 217.

12. Quigley HA, Addicks EM. Regional differences in the structure of the lamina cribrosa and their relation to glaucomatous optic nerve damage. Arch Ophthalmol 1981; 99: 137–143.

13. Dandona L, Quigley HA, Brown AE, Enger C. Quantitative study of optic nerve head capillaries in experimental optic disc pallor. Arch Ophthalmol 1996; 108: 393–398.

14. Armaly NF. Genetic determination of the cup/disc ratio of the optic nerve. Arch Ophthalmol 1967; 68: 401.

15. Carpel EF, Engstrom PF. The normal cup-disc ratio. Am J Ophthalmol 1981; 91: 588.

16. Yablonski ME, Zimmerman TJ, Kass MA, Becker B. Prognostic significance of optic disc cupping in ocular hypertensive patients. Am J Ophthalmol 1980; 89: 585.

17. Yamamoto T, Iwase A, Kawase K, Sawada A, Ishida K. Optic disc hemorrhages detected in a large-scale eye disease screening project. J Glaucoma 2004; 13: 356–60.

18. Soares AS, Artes PH, Andreou P, Leblanc RP, Chauhan BC, Nicolela MT. Factors associated with optic disc hemorrhages in glaucoma. Ophthalmology 2004; 111: 1653–1657.

19. Kono Y, Sugiyama K, Ishida K, Yamamoto T, Kitazawa Y. Characteristics of visual field progression in patients with normal-tension glaucoma with optic disk hemorrhages. Am J Ophthalmol 2003; 135: 499–503.

20. Ahn JK, Park KH. Morphometric change analysis of the optic nerve head in unilateral disk hemorrhage cases. Am J Ophthalmol 2002; 134: 920–922.

21. Ishida K, Yamamoto T, Sugiyama K, Kitazawa Y. Disk hemorrhage is a significantly negative prognostic factor in normal-tension glaucoma. Am J Ophthalmol 2000; 129: 707–714.

22. Jonas JB. Clinical implications of peripapillary atrophy in glaucoma. Curr Opin Ophthalmol 2005; 16: 84–88.

23. Tezel G, Kolker AE, Wax MB, Kass MA, Gordon M, Siegmund KD. Parapapillary chorioretinal atrophy in patients with ocular hypertension. II. An evaluation of progressive changes. Arch Ophthalmol 1997; 115: 1509–1514.

24. Tezel G, Kolker AE, Kass MA, Wax MB, Gordon M, Siegmund KD. Parapapillary chorioretinal atrophy in patients with ocular hypertension. I. An evaluation as a predictive factor for the development of glaucomatous damage. Arch Ophthalmol. 1997; 115: 1503–1508.

25. Uchida H, Ugurlu S, Caprioli J. Increasing peripapillary atrophy is associated with progressive glaucoma. Ophthalmology 1998; 105: 1541–1545.
26. Uhm KB, Lee DY, Kim JT, Hong C. Peripapillary atrophy in normal and primary open-angle glaucoma. Korean J Ophthalmol 1998; 12: 37–50.
27. Sommer A, Quigley HA, Robin AL, *et al*. Evaluation of nerve fiber layer assessment. Arch Ophthalmol 1984; 102: 1766.
28. Airaksinen PJ, Drance SM: Neuroretinal rim area and retinal nerve layer in glaucoma. Arch Ophthalmol 1985; 103: 203.
29. Sommer A, Katz J, Quigley HA, *et al*. Clinically detectable nerve fiber atrophy precedes the onset of glaucomatous field loss. Arch Ophthalmol 1991; 109: 77.
30. Jonas JB, Schiro D. Localised wedge shaped defects of the retinal nerve fibre layer in glaucoma. Br J Ophthalmol 1994; 78: 285–290.
31. Airaksinen PJ, Drance SM. Neuroretinal rim area and retinal nerve fiber layer in glaucoma. Arch Ophthalmol 1985; 103: 203–204.
32. Airaksinen PJ, Tuulonen A. Early glaucoma changes in patients with and without an optic disc haemorrhage. Acta Ophthalmol (Copenh) 1984; 62: 197–202.
33. Quigley HA, Miller NR, George T. Clinical evaluation of nerve fiber layer atrophy as an indicator of glaucomatous optic nerve damage. Arch Ophthalmol 1980; 98: 1564–1571.
34. Sommer A, Miller NR, Pollack I, Maumenee AE, George T. The nerve fiber layer in the diagnosis of glaucoma. Arch Ophthalmol 1977; 95: 2149–2156.

Chapter 8

Imaging technology in the assessment of the optic disc and retinal nerve fiber layer

Why should I read this chapter?

Imaging of the morphology of the optic nerve and nerve fiber layer is an invaluable tool in aiding the clinician looking after the glaucoma or suspect glaucoma patient. All the devices described in this chapter are imperfect tools and in order to use them it is vital that the clinician understands the strengths and weaknesses of each. This chapter will help you decide what tests to use and how to interpret their findings.

Introduction

There are numerous imaging devices available which aim to assess morphology and give the user information as to the normality of the optic disc or nerve fiber layer. *These do not replace clinical examination.* There are many problems associated with such devices and interpretation of the evidence they present may lead to significant errors of judgment. Remember you are treating the patient in front of you and not the numbers on their results. Clinical examination is essential and no amount of clever technology will replace a thorough, methodical and systematic assessment of the disc. Sounds familiar!

We know that more than a third of the RNFL can be lost through glaucoma before any defect is noted on visual-field testing and that changes in the RNFL may precede detectable field loss by up to 6 years.[1]

RNFL examination can be difficult, especially in the older population where the NFL is already diffusely thinned. In this same population there are often media opacities such as cataract or corneal pathology which make the detection of subtle RNFL defects challenging.

Assessment of the optic nerve is also not without its difficulties, which are again compounded by any media opacities. Practice in optic nerve assessment will allow the clinician to pick up subtle changes, but the detection of slight progression is difficult. This is mainly due to problems of documentation and quantification of degree of damage. Naturally if a notch has developed where there was none before then it clear cut that the disc has changed and the glaucoma has worsened. However to get this degree of change, a significant degree of NRR must have been lost. The ability to pick up subtle changes before the clinical examination demonstrates a change is one of the key aims of modern glaucoma imaging devices. By having precise quantification of the morphological state of the nerve head (and nerve fiber layer) one can detect subtle changes early and institute treatment appropriately to prevent visual field loss. This sounds too good to be true and unfortunately it is. If the imaging devices were perfect then this would work but they are far from perfect.

Not only would these devices be able to detect changes in the nerve head and RNFL they would also be able to tell us which eyes are healthy and which are not. One would simply examine a large enough number of normals with the device and then examine a large group of patients with glaucoma and allow the computer to do the rest. With an appropriate normal database you should be able to scan a patient and have a print-out telling you whether they have glaucoma or not. Unfortunately again this is not yet possible. Modern technology has allowed us to image the nerve and RNFL with greater detail and the software can now give us indications of the likelihood of normality versus the likelihood of glaucoma. Again it is not perfect and interpretation of these results without an understanding of the weaknesses of each device will result in mismanagement of the patient. The clinician must use the results cautiously and incorporate them with all the available data (vitally including the clinical examination) to make a diagnosis or a decision on management.

Scanning laser polarimetry (SLP), confocal scanning laser ophthalmoscopy (CSLO) and optical coherence tomography (OCT) are imaging techniques that have been seeing increased use in glaucoma over the last decade. Their clinical use is increasing but so is the danger that those utilizing them are using them inappropriately. Even more worrisome is the fear that some clinicians are using them in place of clinical examination techniques. These imaging modalities are adjuncts and not replacements to the clinician's clinical assessment.

This chapter reviews each of these technologies and provides guidelines for their use in clinical practice as well as highlighting the problems that can be encountered with them. The technicalities of doing the tests are not described here.

In what clinical scenarios would these imaging modalities be helpful?

(1) Screening for glaucoma – taking an at-risk population or a general population and subjecting them to the test in the hope of picking up glaucomas
(2) Identifying progression to glaucoma in at-risk groups such as ocular hypertensives or relatives of glaucoma patients
(3) Differentiating physiological cupping from glaucoma
(4) Quantifying the degree of glaucomatous optic neuropathy
(5) Ensuring stability of glaucoma or detecting progression early with confidence

None of the current devices do any of the above with anything like the precision and consistency we would desire. Variations in the optic discs and RNFL of the normal population make a precise cut-off between abnormal and normal impossible. These tools can easily distinguish severe glaucoma (e.g. a cup of CDR 0.9) from a healthy disc with no cup whatsoever. In such a circumstance they have almost 100% success in making the differentiation. Importantly, however, so can the clinician with simple slit lamp biomicroscopy, a much simpler and cheaper option. When the clinician is in doubt about the appearance of the optic nerve head – is it glaucoma or not? – then the imaging devices also, infuriatingly, struggle to make the differentiation.

It must be remembered that the 'gold standard' to which all of these tools are compared is clinical examination by a glaucoma specialist. These glaucoma specialists have the benefit of knowing the visual fields and the IOP and they have the time to detect progression and thus confirm a diagnosis of glaucoma. They take all the clinical information before making a diagnosis of glaucoma or normality and thus so should you.

The accuracy of any of these devices pales next to the accuracy of a clinician physically examining the patient and taking all the clinical information into account.

The clinician also has the benefit of using the information from the imaging devices and factoring this into the equation. A diagnosis cannot be made on these devices alone. In competent hands, specialized in the management of glaucoma, the utility of these imaging devices is equivocal.

Scanning laser polarimetry

The GDx (Laser Diagnostic Technologies, San Diego, CA) is a scanning laser polarimeter which is designed to measure the thickness of the peripapillary RNFL. We know that the RNFL is lost in glaucoma and that this loss may precede the visual-field loss by a significant amount of time. The GDx measures the RNFL by measuring retardation values.

When polarized light (light waves aligned into only one plane) passes through a thin grating it is forced to rotate its plane of motion to get through this grating. This is called a phase shift and is proportional to the thickness of the grating. If the grating it is passing through is very thick then all the light passing through it undergoes this phase shift to align itself with the microscopic gaps in the grating. In thinner gratings the phase shift is incomplete.

The ability to alter the phase of polarized light is a manifestation of birefringence. The main source of this birefringence in the eye is the RNFL due to the linear orientation of the millions of axons as they sweep in to form the optic nerve. The cornea and, to a much lesser degree, the lens also have birefringent properties. Each eye is different with regard to is corneal birefringence. Previous GDx machines have used fixed corneal compensation (FCC), i.e. they used a generalized calculation to correct for these corneal properties. This led to significant inaccuracies in the measurements, as different eyes have different polarization properties making removal of corneal and lenticular noise impossible.

The modern version of the machine now uses variable corneal compensation (VCC), which is known to significantly improve the ability of the device to distinguish between healthy and glaucomatous eyes.[2,3]

The GDx VCC compensates for the anterior segement birefringence by scanning the macula first. In all eyes the RNFL around the fovea is orientated radially with the axons pointing straight at fixation. All the fibers from the temporal disc run virtually horizontally into the macula. By scanning this area the device sees how much anterior segment noise is present and knows how much to correct the scan by. A subsequent scan of the macula should give a perfect radial pattern thus ensuring that all the polarizing effect of the cornea and lens has been negated. At each subsequent scan the GDx VCC carries out this test again to ensure nothing has changed. It should be able to detect if the patient has had cataract surgery as the macula scan will now not be correct, thus necessitating a further 'calibration scan'. Incorrect compensation will result in a bow-tie pattern in the macula while full compensation will show a uniformly blue scan.

Advantages include:

- Quick – image acquisition time is less than one second
- Mydriasis not required although still works well even if patient dilated[4]
- The test may be performed accurately on patients wearing contact lenses[5], pseudophakes[6], or in silicone oil filled eyes[7]
- Has a large gender-, age-, and ancestry-adjusted normative database (see below)
- Anterior segment surgery should have no effect on the GDx VCC as the inherent nature of the VCC compensates for any such changes in anterior birefringence

Disadvantages include:

- Images may be degraded in patients with corneal diseases, corneal grafts, advanced cataracts, peripapillary and retinal atrophy, high myopia[8]
- Struggles with tilted discs[9,10]
- Split nerve fiber bundles present in approximately 12% of normal subjects can be mistaken for a focal wedge defect associated with glaucoma[11]
- Motion artifacts (which are not detected by the original GDx machine) can increase retardation values in a haphazard manner, especially in glaucoma patients.[12] The newer GDx VCC checks for eye movement, which is highlighted under 'fixation' category on the 'image check screen' after scan acquisition

Normative database

The GDx has a large normative database based upon 540 normal eyes (mean age of 43.9 years) and 271 glaucomatous eyes (mean age of 65.7 years). More than 70% of this group were white people.

Reading the GDx print-out

Check the quality score, it should be above seven.
There are five sets of images given on the printout (Fig. 8.1):

- Fundus image
- Thickness map
- Deviation map
- Temporal superior nasal inferior temporal (TSNIT) graph
- Parameter table

Fundus image (top right and left)

This is a color photograph of the fundus. It is important to check that it is focused, evenly illuminated and that the black ellipse is well centered and accurately follows the rim of the optic disc. This optic disc outline is not vital as it is simply used to calculate the center of the optic

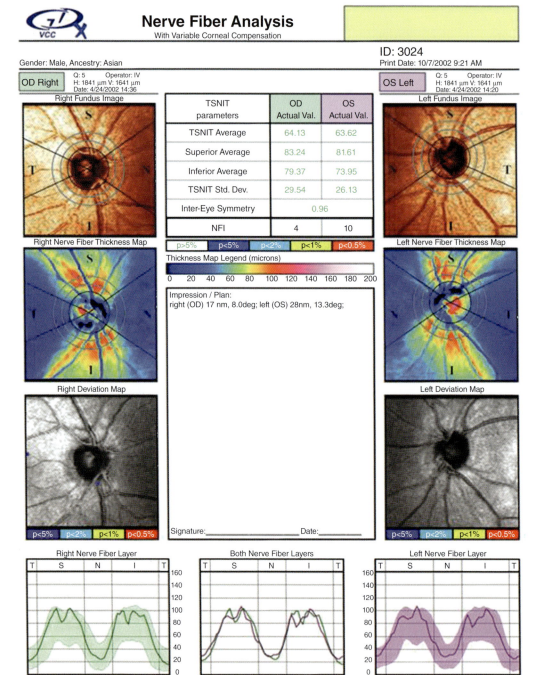

Figure 8.1 GDx normal print-out.

disc rather than used in the calculations. Check the double white ring is of the correct size. Usually the medium size is used, but if the disc is particularly large or there is excessive PPA the larger ring may be used.

Thickness map (below fundus images)

This is a color-coded display showing RNFL thickness. It is physiologically thicker superiorly and inferiorly. Thick areas are highlighted by yellow, orange and red colors, while thin readings are colored dark blue, light blue and green.

Deviation map (below thickness maps)

This plot compares RNFL values with the age-, race- and sex-specific normative database. It highlights areas of abnormality. Degrees of deviation from these normal values are color-coded according to increased likelihood of abnormality from dark blue, light blue, to yellow and then finally to red.

TSNIT graphs (bottom)

This graph shows the variation of thickness of the RNFL through the 360° of the calculation circle. The normal range is highlighted by the green and purple zones (right and left respectively) and shows the characteristic 'double hump' corresponding to the thickest portions of RNFL superiorly and inferiorly. A comparison between the two eyes is displayed centrally.

Parameter table (top center)

This table displays summary RNFL measures from the two eyes and compares these values with the normative database. Normal values are displayed in green but color-coded if abnormal based on probability of abnormality. The TSNIT standard deviation measures the difference between the thickest portions of the RNFL compared to the thinnest. A normal eye will have a high value because of good normal 'humps'. A comparison between the two eyes (inter-eye symmetry, range -1 to +1) is displayed. Normal eyes should usually have good symmetry (0.9). The nerve fiber index (NFI) is supposedly the best overall indicator of the likelihood of normality. NFI is normal if it is between 0 and 30, borderline 31–50 and outside normal limits if above 50. Several studies have confirmed the clinical utility and validity of using NFI as an indicator of the presence of glaucoma.[13–16] Other work has demonstrated this to be a clinically valuable instrument for the detection of glaucoma.[17–19]

Clinical utility of scanning laser polarimetry

This is a good tool to have. It may be argued that the optic disc imagers are simply doing the same job as the clinician in detecting disc morphology whereas the GDx is assessing the RNFL which is notoriously harder to quantify clinically. Unless a deep and definite wedge defect is present in a younger patient it is hard to identify clinically and certainly the clinician cannot hope to quantify the thickness of the remaining RNFL. There is very little data as yet regarding the use of GDx to detect progression, however the data presented in the literature so far regarding the ability to distinguish glaucoma from normality is encouraging. Taking the NFI into account when considering the intrepretation of a suspicious disc is reasonable.

Confocal scanning laser ophthalmoscopy

The Heidelberg Retinal Tomograph (HRT) (Heidelberg Engineering, Heidelberg, Germany) is a scanning laser ophthalmoscope utilizing a confocal scanning diode laser to provide topographic measurements of the optic disc and peripapillary retina.

A laser beam is scanned across the retina and reflected back to a detector. The emitted laser beam passes through a pinhole and the returning beam has to pass through another pinhole before getting to the detector. The outbound beam and inbound beam are focused on the same spot (confocal). The pinholes ensure that any other laser light being reflected from any other points except the point being scanned is excluded from the image. When the focal point matches with a surface (for example the surface of the NRR) the reflection is maximal and one point on the three-dimensional topographic map is created. Points of focus which are posterior or anterior to this surface will have minimal reflectance. Sequential optical sections are generated allowing the whole map to form.

The HRT II acquires up to 64 optical sections in depth intervals of 1/16 inch. The field of view is fixed at 15° with 384 × 384 pixels per image plane, i.e. it generates almost 150 000 height measurements from which the surface map is created. A reflectivity image is created from the surface plot with the deeper areas represented as darkness and the more superficial layers as light. This is not a photograph but is a digital color-coded height map. The scans are done three times and three maps are generated. Each pixel will have three height values attributed to it and the software presents the mean of these as well as the standard deviation (the mean pixel height standard deviation (MPHSD)). Intuitively the closer the three scans are to each other the more reliable the image will be. If the three images deliver vastly different height maps then the validity of the mean scan should be questioned.

Once the scan is complete the operator draws a line manually around the disc and the software calculates stereometric parameters within this ring. Values are presented for the whole disc and for the six predefined sectors.

A reference plane is dropped 50 μm deep to the temporal disc edge. Everything deep to this plane is called the cup and everything above this plane but within the drawn disc boundaries is called the NRR (Fig. 8.2).

Moorfield's regression analysis is used to analyze the data generated by the HRT II. It is inherently flawed by the fact that is is based upon a sample size of only 112 normal white people and 77 with early glaucoma. Eyes included had a refractive error of less than 6 D and a disc size between 1.2 and 2.8 mm². It does not perform well with small discs, large discs or in tilted discs.

Measurements of optic disc stereometric parameters by HRT are highly reproducible.[20] Use of the RNFL-related parameters should be taken cautiously, however, as there can be operator-induced variability in determining the location of the ellipse, and even with experienced operators there can be a fair amount of image acquisition induced variability.[21] Research

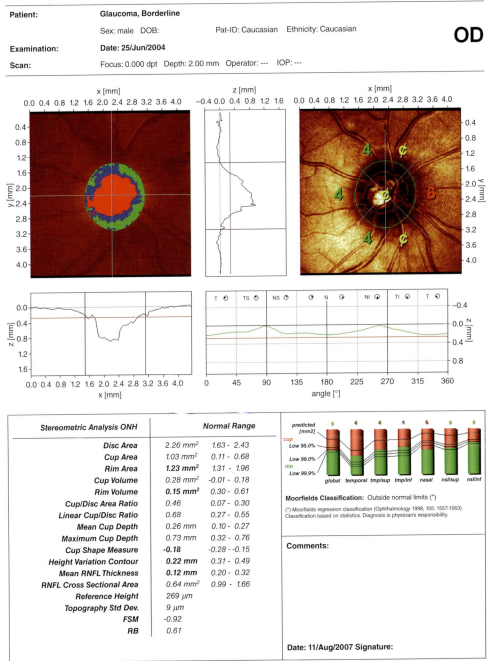

Figure 8.2 HRT II printout.

suggests that there may be a subset of patients with ocular hypertension in whom sequential follow-up with HRT may reveal optic nerve head changes that predate development of glaucomatous field changes.[22]

Advantages of HRT:

- Quick
- No need for mydriasis
- Refractive errors can be compensated for

Disadvantages of HRT:

- All of the calculations are based on the disc drawn by the examiner. This is not always an easy task as the examiner only has the reflectance image to base their judgment of the disc margin on. If the disc is drawn incorrectly all the calculations and analyses are meaningless
- Does not perform well in myopic eyes[23]
- The Moorfield's analysis does not perform well with very small discs or large discs[24,25]

Reading the HRT II report

An initial HRT II printed report is shown in Fig. 8.2.

Topography image (upper left)

The central area represents the cup and is displayed in red. The rim in blue and green, with the green bit being the flat NRR and the blue any area of sloping rim.

Reflection image (upper right)

The optic nerve is shown and divided into six sectors, effectively splitting the disc into six slices of the overall optic disc pie. The rim and the disc area for each sector are compared to a normative database and classified by Moorfield's regression analysis (MRA) as within normal limits (signified by a green tick), borderline (yellow exclamation mark), or outside normal limits (red cross).

Moorfield's regression analysis (bottom right)

This graph shows red and green vertical bars representing the results of MRA. Each column represents the total optic nerve head area for a slice of the pie and is divided into rim area (green) and cup area (red).

Four black lines are drawn across the red/green graph and represent the statistical data of the normative database. The top 'predicted' line marks the point in each sector where 50% of the normal database have a NRR greater than this level. The next line down indicates that 95% of normal discs have a NRR above this point. The next two lines represent the 99.0 and 99.9% levels of NRR size in that sector. If the percentage of the patient's NRR area is above the 95%

limit (i.e. 19 out of 20 of the normal discs in the database had a similar size NRR), then that area is marked with a green tick (within normal limits), between the 95% and 99% lines (i.e. only between 5% and 1% of the normal discs had this area of NRR) it is marked with a yellow exclamation mark (borderline), and finally it is marked with a red cross (outside normal limits) if less than 1% of the normal discs would have such a limited NRR in that sector. This 99% level is the well established statistical level of confidence that that particular area is 'definitely' abnormal.

Table of stereometric analysis of the optic nerve head (bottom left)

This table provides absolute figures and does not present any statistical analysis. The disc size is important as not only will this affect the validity of the MRA but will also have implications on the findings of the clinical examination of the disc. Comparing these absolute values with previous scans may be helpful in considering whether progression has occurred.

Mean height contour graph (middle right)

This plot shows the difference between the red reference line and the green height profile in millimeters and corresponds to the thickness of the RNFL. This measurement is taken for 360° following the disc outline which was drawn by the operator using the reflectance image. This line always starts temporal and rotates clockwise for the right eye and counterclockwise for the left eye. The horizontal red line indicates the location of the reference plane which separates cup and NRR. If the green topography height profile line goes below the red line it indicates that the NRR is below where the cup begins. This is of course impossible and indicates that the contour line was drawn incorrectly in the first place.

Clinical utility of confocal scanning laser ophthalmoscopy

The two most important parts of the HRT II print out are the topography standard deviation and the statement below the Moorfield's regression analysis stating that 'Diagnosis is the clinician's responsibility'.

The topography standard deviation (SD) number (far bottom left of the printout) serves as an image quality control and should be less than 30 to make meaningful interpretation of the scan possible. Scans with a SD far above 30 should be discarded as they will cause confusion, inaccuracies, misdiagnosis and will mess up any attempt to accurately monitor progression.

A follow-up report can be generated after the third scan (the first two scans are used to determine a baseline). Progression analysis is pointless if the quality, and thus reliability, of the scans used are different. One poor-quality scan included in the follow-up may nullify any possible interpretation and fail to give any definitive answer. More worrying is the fact that inclusion and misguided interpretation of such poor scans may mislead the examiner into believing that definite progression has occurred when it is purely artifact.

With the HRT II, the contour line initially drawn is used for all subsequent scans to allow serial analysis. If the disc is drawn incorrectly in the first scan all further scans will have the same error. On the follow-up report, the print-out is always in black and white. Significant changes in topography are displayed in red (where there is NRR loss, i.e. loss of height at that point) or green (increased height).

Recently HRT III software has been produced which is heralded as a significant improvement to the clinical utility of the HRT II. The new software uses an enlarged race-specific database, consisting of eyes of 733 white and 215 Afrocaribbean patients. HRT III software includes the calculation of the glaucoma probability score (GPS), a new, automated algorithm that evaluates both optic disc and peripapillary RNFL topography to provide a probability score of having glaucoma. The GPS uses two measures of peripapillary RNFL shape (horizontal and vertical RNFL curvature) and three measures of optic nerve head shape (cup size, cup depth and rim steepness) to calculate the probability of having damage consistent with glaucoma. One of the major advances in this software is that no contour line is used in the GPS calculation, and therefore the analysis is operator independent. This technique also scrutinizes the normal convex RNFL curvature, caused by the ganglion cell axons forming a slight hump as they bunch together to dip into the optic nerve. As axons are lost as a result of glaucoma this hump inevitably flattens off.

The GPS may be better at detecting patients with early glaucoma (visual field mean deviation of better than −5 dB), with a sensitivity of 72.3% compared with 59.6% for the MRA.[26]

Despite expansion of the normative database, the GPS may still suffer from inaccuracy when faced with large or small optic discs.[27] Early data on the HRT III seems encouraging[28–30] however it has to be emphasized that it is as yet unvalidated and its strengths and weaknesses have not been fully characterized to date.

Ocular coherence tomography

Optical coherence tomography (OCT) (Carl Zeiss Meditec, Dublin, CA) uses a near infrared light to provide cross-sectional images of the optically clear ocular tissues. It is a very similar technology to ultrasound but uses light instead of sound waves to get reflectance information and build up an image of any tissue interfaces it encounters. OCT is based on the principles of low-coherence interferometry.

A low-coherence beam of near infrared light is shone on to a partially reflective mirror. One beam continues through the mirror and enters the eye. The other beam is reflected back. The beam that enters the eye is reflected from the ocular tissues according to their nature, thickness and distance away from the detector. The reflected beam is called the reference beam, while the light that enters the eye forms the measurement beam. Portions of the measurement beam bounce back out of the eye as they come to tissue interfaces and recombine with the reflected beam. When the two beams reunite they interfere with each other. This degree of interference can be detected and is quantifiably related to the retardation of the measurement beam. The delay times of the reflected rays from the various retinal layers are measured and can be translated into an anatomical picture.

Either side of the RNFL there is a transition in tissue structure forming a reflective surface; using this the RNFL thickness may be calculated. OCT has widespread use in assessing macular anatomy, however in glaucoma the major uses are in optic disc assessment and RNFL analysis.

When assessing the optic disc multiple radial linear scans are undertaken to provide cross-sectional data on cupping and NRR. In assessing parapapillary RNFL a single circular scan is taken at a radius of 1.7 mm from the centre of the ONH. This circular scan is unwound and then presented as a linear result. RNFL thickness is presented for superior, inferior, nasal and temporal quadrants and for each clock hour. Mean RNFL thickness is also calculated. Just like the inferior NRR is the most sensitive site for glaucoma damage at the nerve, the inferior RNFL parameter on OCT is the one most strongly associated with glaucoma status.[31–33]

OCT RNFL normative database

The normative database is based upon data from 328 patients with a mean age of 47 years. Of these patients, 63% were white and only 8% were of black ancestry.

RNFL scan

Several analysis protocols can be used for evaluation:

- RNFL thickness – graphs of RNFL thickness along circle scans made around the disc
- RNFL thickness average – RNFL thickness graphs averaged over multiple circle scans of equal radius around the disc. Probably the most useful single scan plot for clinical use
- RNFL thickness map – two maps for each eye of RNFL thickness in an annular region around the disc
- RNFL thickness change – to assess change in RNFL over time between two scans
- RNFL thickness serial analysis – analyzes up to four comparative scans

RNFL thickness average analysis

This scan (Fig. 8.3) allows comparison to the normative database and is probably the most clinically useful. It has both eyes on it, allowing comparison between the two and it also compares each eye to normal data.

RNFL print-out

The top third presents information regarding the right eye, the middle third the left eye and the lower portion further numerical information on both eyes with some statistical analysis.

The RNFL thickness chart is plotted showing the line of RNFL thickness in a TSNIT format. This represents the unwrapped circumferential scan starting temporally, moving round to superiorly then nasally, then inferiorly and finally back full circle to the temporal portion of the RNFL.

Once the normative data software update is incorporated this plot shows the normal ranges by color-coded portions. The green area is the normal area indicating that 90% of all normals fall within this zone. Five percent of the normal population will have a RNFL within or below the yellow zone. Once the plot dips into the red zone it is indicative of statistical confidence of abnormality (only 1% of normals have RNFL readings in this zone).

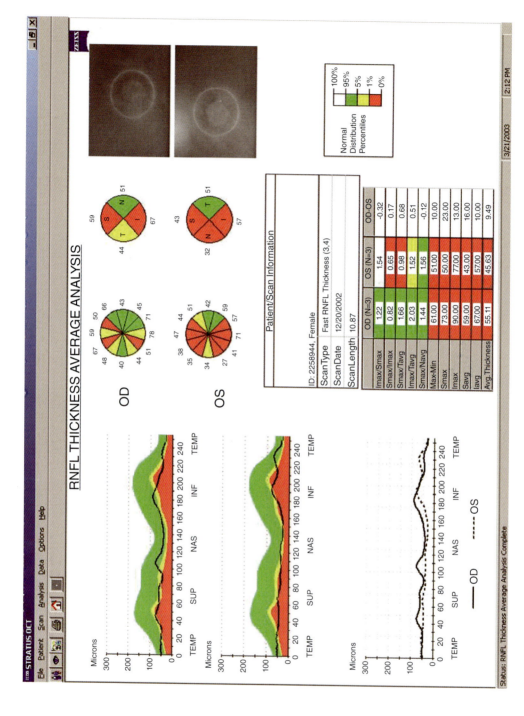

Figure 8.3 OCT RNFL print-out.

Sector and quadrant RNFL thickness averages are presented in the pie-chart type displays to the right of the TSINT plots. On the right of these are the fundus image (used to confirm that the scan is in the right place) and the worst of the scans (to give a visual indication to the examiner of the quality of the scan).

As with the disc OCT a quality indicator is given. Scans with a quality of less than 5 should be discarded. Look upon scans with a quality of less than 7 with slight skepticism, certainly if you are trying to detect progression. The higher the scan quality the better.

The comparative chart allows direct comparison between the RNFL thickness between the two eyes. A table in the bottom right displays the data for each eye and compares numerically between the two.

Optic disc scan

The OCT scan detects the RPE layer and the software analyzes this and decides where the RPE ends. It takes this point as the edge of the disc. It also looks at the RNFL and works out where it bends over to dip into the edge of the cup. Using these two features it calculates cross-sectional information about the cup and the disc.

Optic nerve head analysis report print-out

The print-out is shown in Fig. 8.4.

Individual radial scan analysis (top half)

This scan refers to only one linear scan across the nerve. The orientation of this scan is displayed in the compass-type display in the bottom right of this section. It is set to the vertical by default hopefully assessing the vertical cup–disc dimensions and both superior and inferior poles of the nerve. The parameters displayed on the right show:

- Rim area: this is the NRR area on one side of the radial scan (indicated by the arrow) is calculated
- Average nerve width at disc: the average of nerve bundle widths at each side
- Disc diameter and cup diameter
- Rim length: this is disc diameter minus cup diameter

Naturally the higher the signal strength is the better, but any figure below 5 is worthless. In order to truly assess change then consistent scan qualities of over 7 should be aimed for. A scan with a quality less than 5 should be discarded.

Optic nerve head analysis result (lower half)

Information for this portion is taken from all six radial scans:

- Vertical integrated rim area – this is the average rim area from the six scans multiplied by the disc circumference

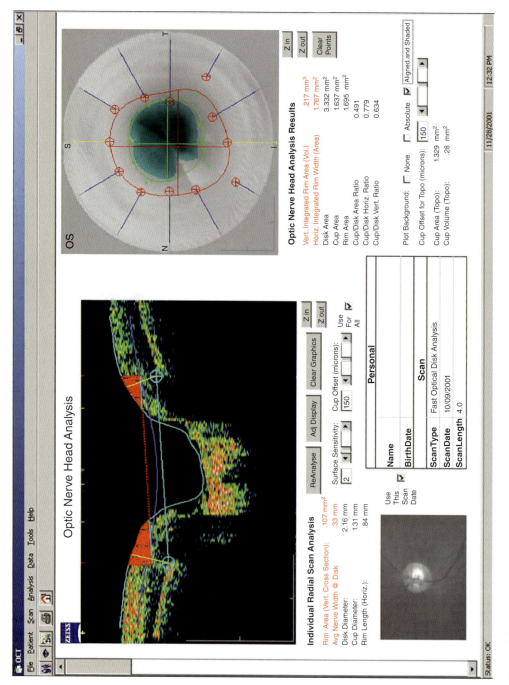

Figure 8.4 OCT disc print-out.

Table 8.1 Advantages and disadvantages of ocular coherence tomography.

Advantages of OCT	Disadvantages of OCT
• Quick • Data are highly reproducible[34] • Tends to correspond with visual-field loss • May work well in tilted discs where other imaging devices may fail[35] • Results tend to be quite reproducible[36]	• Dilatation is required • This is an optical technique and so is highly sensitive to media opacity such as cataract[36]

• Horizontal integrated rim width – this is the average rim width multiplied by the disc circumference

Disc, cup and rim area are displayed as well as maximum horizontal and vertical CDRs. Below this is displayed information on 'Cup offset for topo'. This is set at 150 μm and is the distance anterior to where the RPE ends used for the calculations below it. Imagine filling the disc with water up to this level to give the readings for cup area and cup volume.

Clinical utility of ocular coherence tomography

Advantages and disadvantages of OCT are shown in Table 8.1.

The OCT with the normative database can detect localized RNFL defects with moderate sensitivity and high specificity, and shows good diagnostic agreement with red-free RNFL photographs.[37] Preliminary data suggests that RNFL OCT it is a good tool for discriminating glaucoma from normality.[38][40]

Newer OCT devices are becoming available which have much higher resolution capabilities which will hopefully improve sensitivity and allow more accurate measures of RNFL thickness.

There is very little data regarding the use of the disc OCT protocol and clinically its use is limited.

Which device is best?

None of the devices will work in isolation in diagnosing glaucoma, monitoring for progression or for screening. They all have their inherent weaknesses and strengths. One device may diagnose glaucoma while another may miss it. The other device may pick up a glaucoma which is missed by other devices. Many studies have looked at the devices and compared them head to head, finding no real difference between them with regard to clinical utility in glaucoma.[41–46] They are only as good as the quality of results they produce and the clinician interpreting them.

Interpreting the results of these tests without looking at the disc and RNFL layer yourself and taking it all in context of the other findings is dangerous and will lead to misdiagnosis and mismanagement.

Which device is best? It would be nice to use them all, however this is not possible for the majority of clinicians due to cost and logistics. Any one of the devices will add to the clinical picture and help the clinician make decisions. If the intention is to use the device to spare you assessing the nerve then don't. It is an adjunct to your clinical examination not a replacement.

Newer devices and newer software require the test of time before a definitive judgment can be made.

References

1. Quigley HA, Miller NR, Robin AL, *et al.* Clinically detectable nerve fiber atrophy precedes the onset of glaucomatous field loss. Arch Opthalmol 1991; 77–83.
2. Bagga H, Greenfield DS, Feuer W, Knighton RW. Scanning laser polarimetry with variable corneal compensation and optical coherence tomography in normal and glaucomatous eyes. Am J Ophthalmol 2003; 135(4): 521–529.
3. Brusini P, Salvetat ML, Parisi L, Zeppieri M, Tosoni C. Discrimination between normal and early glaucomatous eyes with scanning laser polarimeter with fixed and variable corneal compensator settings. Eur J Ophthalmol 2005; 15: 468–476.
4. Horani A, Frenkel S, Blumenthal EZ. The effect of pupil dilation on scanning laser polarimetry with variable corneal compensation. Ophthalmic Surg Lasers Imaging 2006; 37: 212–216.
5. Bhandari A, Chen PP, Mills RP. Effects of contact lenses on scanning laser polarimetry of the peripapillary retinal nerve fiber layer. Am J Opthalmol 1999; 127: 722–724.
6. Collur S, Carooll AM, Cameron BD. Human lens effect on in vivo scanning laser polarimetric measurements of retinal nerve fiber layer thickness. Opthalmic Surg Lasers 2000; 2: 126–130.
7. Hollo G, Bereczki A, Milibak T, Suveges I. Scanning laser polarimetry via intravitreal silicone oil. Acta Opthalmol Scand 1999; 77: 519–521.
8. Hoh ST, Greenfield DS, Leibmann JM, *et al.* Factors affecting image acquisition during scanning laser polarimetry. Opthalmic Surg Lasers 1998; 29: 545–551.
9. Bozkurt B, Irkec M, Tatlipinar S, *et al.* Retinal nerve fiber analysis and interpretation of GDx® parameters in patients with tilted disc syndrome. Opthalmol 2001; 24(1): 27–31.
10. Yu S, Tanabe T, Hangai M, Morishita S, Kurimoto Y, Yoshimura N. Scanning laser polarimetry with variable corneal compensation and optical coherence tomography in tilted disk. Am J Ophthalmol 2006; 142: 475–482.
11. Colen TP, Lemij HG. Prevalence of split nerve fiber layer bundles in healthy eyes imaged with scanning laser polarimetry. Opthalmology 2001; 108: 151–156.
12. Colen TP, Lemij HG. Motion artifacts in scanning laser polarimetry. Ophthalmology 2002; 109: 1568–1572.
13. Iester M, Perdicchi A, De Feo F, Fiesoletti E, Amodeo S, Sanna G, Leonardi A, Calabria G. Comparison between GDx VCC parameter and achromatic perimetry in glaucoma patients. J Glaucoma 2006; 15: 281–285.
14. Da Pozzo S, Fuser M, Vattovani O, Di Stefano G, Ravalico G. GDx-VCC performance in discriminating normal from glaucomatous eyes with early visual field loss. Graefes Arch Clin Exp Ophthalmol 2006; 244: 689–695.
15. Da Pozzo S, Iacono P, Marchesan R, Fantin A, Ravalico G. Scanning laser polarimetry with variable corneal compensation and detection of glaucomatous optic neuropathy. Graefes Arch Clin Exp Ophthalmol 2005; 243: 774–779.
16. Reus NJ, Lemij HG. Diagnostic Accuracy of the GDxVCC for Glaucoma. Ophthalmology 2004; 111: 1860–1865.

17. Shaikh A, Salmon JF. The role of scanning laser polarimetry using the GDx variable corneal compensator in the management of glaucoma suspects. Br J Ophthalmol 2006; 90: 1454–1457.
18. Tsai JC, Chang HW, Teng MC, Lin PW, Lai IC. Scanning laser polarimetry for measurement of retinal nerve fiber layer in absolute, advanced and early glaucoma. Chang Gung Med J 2006; 29: 162–168.
19. Munkwitz S, Funk J, Loeffler KU, Harbarth U, Kremmer S. Sensitivity and specificity of scanning laser polarimetry using the GDx. Br J Ophthalmol 2004; 88: 1142–1145.
20. Owen VM, Strouthidis NG, Garway-Heath DF, Crabb DP. Measurement variability in Heidelberg Retina Tomograph imaging of neuroretinal rim area. Invest Ophthalmol Vis Sci 2006; 47: 5322–5330.
21. Miglior S, Albe E, Guareschi M, et al. Intra-observer and inter-observer reproducibility in the evaluation of optic disc stereometric parameter by Heidelberg Retina Tomograph. Opthalmology 2002; 109: 1072–1077.
22. Kamal DS, Garway-Heath DF, Hitchings RA, Fitzke FW. Use of sequential Heidelberg Retina Tomograph images to identify changes at the optic disc in ocular hypertensive patients at risk of developing glaucoma. Br J Opthalmol 2000; 84: 993–998.
23. Yamazaki Y, Yoshikawa K, Kunimatsu S, et al. Influence of myopic disc shape on the diagnostic precision of the Heidelberg Retina Tomograph. Jpn J Opthalmol 1999; 43: 392–397.
24. Hawker MJ, Vernon SA, Ainsworth G. Specificity of the Heidelberg Retina Tomograph's diagnostic algorithms in a normal elderly population: the Bridlington Eye Assessment Project. Ophthalmology 2006; 113: 778–785.
25. Girkin CA, DeLeon-Ortega JE, Xie A, McGwin G, Arthur SN, Monheit BE. Comparison of the Moorfields classification using confocal scanning laser ophthalmoscopy and subjective optic disc classification in detecting glaucoma in blacks and whites. Ophthalmology 2006; 113: 2144–2149.
26. Harizman N, Zelefsky JR, Ilitchev E, Tello C, Ritch R, Liebmann JM. Detection of glaucoma using operator-dependent versus operator-independent classification in the Heidelberg retinal tomograph-III. Br J Ophthalmol 2006; 90: 1390–1392.
27. Coops A, Henson DB, Kwartz AJ, Artes PH. Automated analysis of Heidelberg retina tomograph optic disc images by glaucoma probability score. Invest Ophthalmol Vis Sci 2006; 47: 5348–5355.
28. Harizman N, Zelefsky JR, Ilitchev E, Tello C, Ritch R, Liebmann JM. Heidelberg retinal tomograph-III. Br J Ophthalmol 2006; 90: 1390–1392.
29. Burgansky-Eliash Z, Wollstein G, Bilonick RA, Ishikawa H, Kagemann L, Schuman JS. Glaucoma detection with the Heidelberg Retina Tomograph 3. Ophthalmology 2006 [Epub ahead of print].
30. Zelefsky JR, Harizman N, Mora R, Ilitchev E, Tello C, Ritch R, Liebmann JM. Assessment of a race-specific normative HRT-III database to differentiate glaucomatous from normal eyes. J Glaucoma 2006; 15: 548–551.
31. Guedes V, Schuman JS, Hertzmark MA, et al. Optical coherence tomography measurement of macular and nerve fiber layer thickness in normal and glaucomatous human eyes. Opthalmology 2003; 110: 177–189.
32. Chen HY, Wang TH, Lee YM, Hung TJ. Retinal nerve fiber layer thickness measured by optical coherence tomography and its correlation with visual-field defects in early glaucoma. J Formos Med Assoc 2005; 104: 927–934.
33. Sihota R, Sony P, Gupta V, Dada T, Singh R. Diagnostic capability of optical coherence tomography in evaluating the degree of glaucomatous retinal nerve fiber damage. Invest Ophthalmol Vis Sci 2006; 47: 2006–2010.
34. Blumenthal EZ, Williams JM, Weinreb RN, et al. Reproducibility of nerve fiber layer thickness measurements by use of optical coherence tomography. Opthalmology 2000; 107: 2278–2282.
35. Yu S, Tanabe T, Hangai M, Morishita S, Kurimoto Y, Yoshimura N. Scanning laser polarimetry with variable corneal compensation and optical coherence tomography in tilted disk. Am J Ophthalmol 2006; 142: 475–482.

36. Budenz DL, Chang RT, Huang X, Knighton RW, Tielsch JM. Reproducibility of retinal nerve fiber thickness measurements using the stratus OCT in normal and glaucomatous eyes. Invest Ophthalmol Vis Sci 2005; 46: 2440–2443.
36. Savini G, Zanini M, Barboni P. Influence of pupil size and cataract on retinal nerve fiber layer thickness measurements by Stratus OCT. J Glaucoma 2006; 15: 336–340.
37. Jeoung JW, Park KH, Kim TW, Khwarg SI, Kim DM. Diagnostic ability of optical coherence tomography with a normative database to detect localized retinal nerve fiber layer defects. Ophthalmology 2005; 112: 2157–2163.
38. Anton A, Moreno-Montanes J, Blazquez F, Alvarez A, Martin B, Molina B. Usefulness of optical coherence tomography parameters of the optic disc and the retinal nerve fiber layer to differentiate glaucomatous, ocular hypertensive, and normal eyes. J Glaucoma 2007; 16: 1–8.
39. Lalezary M, Medeiros FA, Weinreb RN, Bowd C, Sample PA, Tavares IM, Tafreshi A, Zangwill LM. Baseline optical coherence tomography predicts the development of glaucomatous change in glaucoma suspects. Am J Ophthalmol 2006; 142: 576–582.
40. Budenz DL, Michael A, Chang RT, McSoley J, Katz J. Sensitivity and specificity of the StratusOCT for perimetric glaucoma. Ophthalmology 2005; 112: 3–9.
41. Medeiros FA, Zangwill LM, Bowd C, Weinreb RN. Comparison of the GDX VCC Scanning Laser Polarimeter, HRT Confocal Scanning Laser Ophthalmoscope and Stratus OCT Optical Coherence Tomograph for the detection of glaucoma. Arch Ophthalmol 2004: 122: 827–837.
42. Greaney MJ, Hoffman DC, Garway-Heath DF, et al. Comparison of optic nerve imaging methods to distinguish normal eyes from those with glaucoma. Invest Ophthalmol Visual Sciences 2002: 43: 140–145.
43. Brusini P, Salvetat ML, Zeppieri M, Tosoni C, Parisi L, Felletti M. Comparison between GDx VCC scanning laser polarimetry and Stratus OCT optical coherence tomography in the diagnosis of chronic glaucoma. Acta Ophthalmol Scand 2006; 84: 650–655.
44. Deleon-Ortega JE, Arthur SN, McGwin G Jr, Xie A, Monheit BE, Girkin CA. Discrimination between glaucomatous and nonglaucomatous eyes using quantitative imaging devices and subjective optic nerve head assessment. Invest Ophthalmol Vis Sci 2006; 47: 3374–3380.
45. Bowd C, Zangwill LM, Medeiros FA, Tavares IM, Hoffmann EM, Bourne RR, Sample PA, Weinreb RN. Structure-function relationships using confocal scanning laser ophthalmoscopy, optical coherence tomography, and scanning laser polarimetry. Invest Ophthalmol Vis Sci 2006; 47: 2889–2895.
46. Kanamori A, Nagai-Kusuhara A, Escano MF, Maeda H, Nakamura M, Negi A. Comparison of confocal scanning laser ophthalmoscopy, scanning laser polarimetry and optical coherence tomography to discriminate ocular hypertension and glaucoma at an early stage. Graefes Arch Clin Exp Ophthalmol 2006; 244: 58–68.

Chapter 9

The intraocular pressure

Why should I read this chapter?

Numerical IOP is not the be-all and end-all of glaucoma. Taking IOP as the sole criterion for glaucoma will miss a significant number of people with glaucomatous optic neuropathy at normal pressures (NTG) and lead to over-treatment and misdiagnosis of normal people with raised pressures (OHT). In addition, our gold standard of IOP measurement is becoming recognized as being inherently flawed necessitating input on the clinician's part in interpreting IOP findings.

Measuring IOP

The distribution of intraocular pressure (IOP) in populations aged 20–40 years with no known eye disease resembles a normal, or gaussian, distribution (bell-shaped curve with the mean in the middle) but has a skew towards the right (i.e. towards higher pressures).[1] The adult mean IOP is 15.5 mmHg with a standard deviation of 2.6 mmHg. In a normally distributed data set the range of normality is the mean plus or minus 2 standard deviations making the normal range of pressures approximating 10–21 mmHg with theoretically 97.5% of the normal population lying within these limits. This data is based upon measurements utilizing applanation tonometry. It is not quite so simple, however, because of the skew in the distribution of the IOPs making precise definition of the upper limit of normal IOP very difficult.

The IOP is one of several risk factors for development of glaucomatous optic neuropathy. Some patients may develop optic neuropathy at normal pressures whereas conversely some patients may have IOPs above the normal range and never develop any optic neuropathy or visual-field loss in their lifetime. Although the IOP is not a definitive method of differentiating between glaucoma and normality it is still of paramount importance to obtain accurate and reproducible measurements. In addition to facilitating diagnosis of glaucoma it also allows assessment of treatment efficacy. It is becoming accepted that the IOP readings obtained may not actually represent the true pressure inside the eye. An awareness of this fact is vital as it may prevent false perception of treatment success.

Tonometry

Tonometry is based upon simple principles. The higher the pressure in a sphere (whatever its nature) the greater the force required to indent it. Higher pressure will mean that the sphere is firm and a fixed force applied externally will indent it less than if the sphere is softer. Conversely in order to create a certain level of indentation more external force will have to be applied to the firmer sphere.

Clinical tonometry measures IOP by quantifying the deformation of the globe to the force responsible for this deformation. Eyes are usually subjected to a force which results in deformation and flattening of the cornea either by contact from the tonometer apparatus or by non-contact force applied by a stream of propelled air.

At present the clinician managing the glaucoma patient has to be confident in Goldmann applanation tonometry (GAT). Despite its weaknesses it remains the most consistent and clinically relevant measurement of IOP in clinical practice. In the future other techniques may come to the forefront and supercede GAT but for the foreseeable future its measurement remains vital in glaucoma management.

Applanation tonometry

Applanation tonometry measures IOP by subjecting the eye to a known force that flattens the cornea. The most widely used and reliable method is the Goldmann applanation tonometer.

Goldmann applanation tonometer

The basic theory behind GAT is based upon the Imbert–Fick principle. Basically this relies on the fact that when a flat surface is applanated against the cornea causing flattening, the pressure in the eye may be calculated by the force applied divided by the area of contact.

Goldmann worked out that a circular surface of 3.06 mm diameter should be used to applanate the cornea in order to balance the elastic repulsive force of the cornea against the attractive force of the capillary action of the tear film. The grams of force applied to cause flattening is multiplied by a factor of ten to give a reading in millimeters of mercury. All of these calculations were based upon a corneal thickness of 520 μm (0.52 mm). It is now widely accepted that there may be systematic errors associated with IOP measurement using GAT in patients with thicker or thinner corneas than the 'standard' 520 μm. This is now an important feature of glaucoma management and warrants its own chapter (see Chapter 10).

The GAT consists of a plastic biprism on a metal rod attached to a coiled spring which can be adjusted to change the forward force of the biprism head. Fluorescein stain is applied to the anesthetized cornea. The GAT is mounted on a slit lamp and aligned so that the examiner looks down the barrel of the biprism. Cobalt blue light is shone on to the eye/tip of the biprism and the tip is slowly advanced to make contact with the cornea. Two semicircles are seen due to the image of the tear film meniscus surrounding the head being split into two by the biprism. The dial is now adjusted to alter the forward force of the biprism while it remains in contact with the cornea. The semicircles will move when the dial is altered, and when the inner margins (Fig. 9.1) of the two semicircles just touch, the applanation area reaches exactly 3.06 mm in diameter. The force used can then be measured off the knob and simply multiplied by 10 to give a millimeters of mercury IOP reading. Advantages and disadvantages of Goldmann applanation tonometry and sources of inaccuracies are given below (Box 9.1 and 9.2).

For full technique see Appendix.

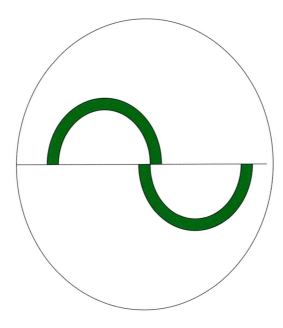

Figure 9.1 Semicircles for GAT IOP measurement. Diagram showing exact end-point for Goldmann applanation tonometry measurement. The fluorescent semicircles should just meet at their inner aspect. Care should be taken to ensure the semicircles are not too thin or too wide.

Box 9.1 Advantages and disadvantages of Goldmann applanation tonometry.

Advantages
Reliable
Current 'gold standard'
Little intra- and inter-observer variability
Independent of scleral rigidity
Easy to master
Highly reproducible

Disadvantages
Unreliable on markedly abnormal corneas such as in cases of corneal edema
Inaccurate on thicker or thinner corneas
Concerns about infection with reusable tonometer heads

Perkins applanation tonometer

The Perkins applanation tonometer is a portable, forehead-supported version of the GAT. It uses the same principles as the GAT and uses an almost identical biprism. It is portable and

Box 9.2 Sources of inaccuracies.

Overestimates of true IOP
Examiner pressing on globe while holding lids open
Wide semicircle meniscus
Unequal biprism semicircles due to misalignment
Increased corneal curvature/marked astigmatism
Thicker cornea
Patient squeezing due to apprehension
Valsalva maneuver – patient holding their breath and increasing venous pressure and thus IOP

Underestimates
Semicircle meniscus too thin/not enough fluorescein on ocular surface
Pathological corneal thickening such as in corneal edema
Previous ocular massage such as gonioscopy
Carotid occlusive disease
Thinner corneas

can thus be used for patients who cannot get up to the slit lamp. The measurement end-point is the same as in GAT but the technique is trickier and thus more liable to variability. It does not replace GAT.

Non-contact tonometry

Again the principles of this technique are identical to those of the GAT. Instead of using a contact method to applanate the cornea, the non-contact methods use the force generated by a puff of air to flatten the cornea. The force of the air is increased until a fixed area of the cornea is flattened. This reading is used to calculate the IOP.

There are many different devices available however they all use similar principles. The device is aligned on the cornea. A collimated light is projected on to the corneal apex. A detector/sensor sits in the same device and detects these rays as they are reflected from the cornea. A pneumatic system produces a puff of air focused at the corneal apex where the collimated light is aimed. The force of the air puff increases in a linear fashion until the cornea is flattened. At this point the light projected on to the flat cornea bounces directly into the detector thus triggering the end-point. The force of air is read and converted to an IOP measurement.

The measurement takes milliseconds and thus there may be variability between different readings as the eye is 'caught' at different parts of the ocular pulse. Repeated readings on the same eye with non-contact tonometry produce a variability of up to 10 mmHg.[2] Several averaged readings are thus required to ensure accurate readings.

The CCT Issue

As previously described CCT has a significant effect on the accuracy of IOP readings. There are several new devices which have been developed in the hope of overcoming this CCT confounding factor and giving a true indication of the IOP. The clinical relevance of 'true' IOP measurement has not been fully characterized, however it makes intuitive sense that in a pressure-dependent disease it is helpful to understand the true pressure within the eye. Certainly the theoretical role of this in patients with an apparently 'normal' IOP by GAT cannot be underestimated. The new devices and the clinical relevance and utility of these devices are detailed in Chapter 10.

Diurnal variation of IOP

It is important to recognize that IOP is not static. As with many biological functions there is some diurnal variation throughout the day and night. In normal eyes, daily fluctuations in measured IOP can change by up to 6 mmHg. In eyes with glaucoma, this diurnal pattern is exaggerated with reported fluctuations of up to 30 mmHg in extreme cases.[3]

The daily cycle of IOP variation generally follows a reproducible pattern, with the maximum IOP in the early or midmorning[3] and the minimum IOP measured late at night. With this information it would make sense that the IOP reading should always be taken at the midmorning time point to catch the peak of IOP. It is this peak which is clinically significant as it has been demonstrated that significant fluctuations in IOP may be related to glaucoma progression. Unfortunately it is not so simple and there are patients who may have an altered diurnal curve of IOP.[4] Some individuals have an IOP peak in the afternoon or evening, and others follow no consistent pattern.[5] Thus a single IOP measurement in the morning may miss a patient's peak pressure and normal IOPs measured at this time may miss significant late spikes of IOP.

The cause for this diurnal IOP fluctuation is thought to be changes in aqueous production rather than alterations in aqueous outflow. Brubaker has established, through fluorophotometry (a technique whereby aqueous production is measured by dilution of fluorescein concentration over time in the AC), that the rate of aqueous humor production is lowest during sleep and increases dramatically just before waking, thus explaining the higher IOP in most people in the morning.[6] Brubaker[6] suggests that circulating catecholamines, specifically epinephrine, may be responsible for this diurnal variation of aqueous production.

One study showed that half of IOP peaks occurred at times outside of normal working hours and that more elevated readings occurred in patients with suspected or documented progression of glaucomatous damage.[7] Another study looking at NTG patients,[8] found that in about 5% of their patients the IOPs breached out of normality and the patients were subsequently reclassified as POAG. Peak IOP readings were obtained outside clinic hours (1800–0800) in 41.4% of these patients.

Importance of IOP fluctuation

Assuming the patient has pressure-dependent disease it is reasonable to theorize that the higher the IOP the worse the ensuing damage. This damage–IOP relationship is not linear however. A patient who sustains damage at a rate of, for example, 1 dB of visual-field loss per month at an IOP of 25 mmHg will not sustain double the rate of damage with a sustained IOP of 50 mmHg. Of course the rate of damage will be much greater at this higher level of IOP. The graph of damage–IOP is probably more similar to an exponential curve.

If we take an IOP at which the patient does not progress (effectively their target IOP, see Chapter 15) then the rate of damage is probably proportional to the IOP above this level squared or maybe even cubed. There is no scientific evidence to support this argument, but it is intuitive and backed by clinical experience. The exact figures are not important, however the concept of the non-linear relationship is vital. For example, if a patient has never progressed with an IOP below 15 mmHg it may be theorized that the patient will progress four times faster at a consistent pressure of 25 mmHg compared to a pressure of 20 mmHg. At a pressure of 20 mmHg (5 above target) the theoretical rate of progression would be $5^2 = 25$ arbitrary progression units. At an IOP of 25 mmHg (10 above target) the rate of progression would be $10^2 = 100$ arbitrary progression units.

Essentially, the closer we get to target IOP the slower the rate of progression. This is obvious, but it does not take into account the diurnal curve. The higher the IOP in the day and the longer this high IOP is maintained, the greater the likelihood and rapidity of progression.

In Fig. 9.2 it can be seen that the patient's IOP fluctuates significantly. When the IOP peaks above the safe IOP damage starts to occur. The damage will occur slowly within the yellow zone and will occur much faster within the red zone. The longer the patient is in the red zone the greater the risk and rapidity of progression. It is important that such IOP spikes into the danger zone are prevented or minimized. It is impossible to appreciate this unless the patient's diurnal curve is, if not formally assessed, at least contemplated and understood.

Measuring the diurnal curve

In the great majority of patients measurement of the diurnal curve is not required. The majority of IOP assessments should be in the morning in order to pick up the highest point on the

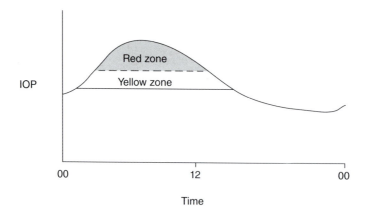

Figure 9.2 Diagram showing an example of a patient's diurnal IOP variation. In the morning the IOP is high enough to cause glaucomatous damage.

IOP curve of most patients. In addition all such measurements should have a time of day documented. The target pressure in any patient should be specific to a certain time range and thus a particular portion of the patient's diurnal curve. If the patient's clinician only has clinics in the afternoon then the target pressures set at that clinic attendance will refer to target pressures for further afternoon clinics (see Chapter 15). The situation is more complex when attempting to make a diagnosis of glaucoma or managing glaucoma suspects, as the 'normal' IOP may give inappropriate reassurance. There is the potential that the patient with the habitually normal IOPs each afternoon has a markedly high IOP at 9 am each day – a raised IOP which is consistently missed.

Logistically, most clinicians will not have the facilities available to measure 24-hour IOP. In most patients, however, it is possible to undertake day phasing of IOP during 'office hours' and hopefully slightly beyond. In the hospital setting there is usually someone available (be they nurse practitioner or junior doctor) who is capable of GAT. Ideally the patient should have their IOP measured and documented by the same individual using the same technique every 2 hours from 6 am to 10 pm (daytime phasing). In reality measurements between 8 am and 6 pm (office hour phasing) is a more realistic proposition and should provide the clinician with a reasonable interpretation of the patient's diurnal curve. If the facilities are not available for even office hour phasing then the clinician may determine information regarding the patient's diurnal IOP pattern from sequential clinic visits. A patient may attend for a 9 am clinic appointment on one occasion, then attend a midday clinic appointment at their first follow-up and then 4 pm for their third visit. This would allow a reasonable although not exhaustive idea of their IOP change during the day. Naturally such sporadic visiting times will make it extremely difficult to judge treatment efficacy. If treatment is commenced at the first visit (9 am measurement) and the patient is reassessed at their second visit (midday) and found to have sustained a pressure reduction it is impossible to determine whether this pressure reduction was due to the treatment or simply due to the fact that the patient was reassessed at another (lower) point on their diurnal IOP profile. It is important that the IOP taken after commencement of treatment is at the same time as the pre-treatment IOP assessment.

This potential clinical uncertainty highlights the need to document the time of IOP measurement at every clinical visit and appreciate that any apparent differences may be due to diurnal fluctuation.

Clinical scenario

Patient seen with IOP of 18 mmHg at 4 pm. Commenced on treatment. Reviewed again 2 months later at 10 am. IOP now 17 mmHg. Are the drops working?

It appears not; had the patient's diurnal curve been plotted at each visit, however, the results may have been as shown in Table 9.1. Thus the patient's whole curve has been lowered *but* the readings were taken at different points on the patient's daily IOP pattern (bold readings).

When to phase patients

Phasing is a valuable tool[9] which should be available in some form to all glaucoma clinicians.

Table 9.1 Phased intraocular pressure reading for patient in clinical scenario.

Time	Pre-treatment visit	Post-treatment visit
8 am	26	18
10 am	23	**17**
12 midday	20	15
2 pm	18	14
4 pm	**18**	14
6 pm	17	13

Normal-tension glaucoma

Also see Chapter 20.

A diagnosis of NTG should not be made without first assessing the patient's diurnal curve. There are patients who will have a normal IOP on repeated measurements but spike up to high levels at another part of the day. Why is this important? If you are going to treat the patient anyway then why bother assessing their diurnal curve?

If you see a patient with an IOP of 14 mmHg and a suspicious disc then you may consider treatment. The decision to treat will be dictated by many patient factors, such as the degree of optic disc cupping or the presence of any visual-field defect. IOP will inevitably play a role in the decision to make a diagnosis of NTG and will certainly be a factor when considering treatment. Knowing that the IOP actually increases to supranormal levels (above 22 mmHg) or even closer to the upper limit of normal may make the diagnosis easier and also dictate a greater tendency to commencing IOP-lowering treatment.

The diagnosis of NTG is arbitrary and there are many different diagnostic criteria in use with different IOP cut-off points to make this diagnosis. It is counterintuitive to see a patient with an IOP consistently of 21 mmHg (thereby labelling them as NTG) and expect them to behave in a different clinical manner to a patient with an IOP of 23 mmHg and a label of POAG. These patients probably have pressure-dependent disease and they both will respond in the same way to IOP lowering. Just because we have put a line in the sand at 21 or 22 mmHg it does not mean that these two patients have different causes for their glaucoma. They may indeed have differing corneal thicknesses meaning that they actually have a similar 'true' IOP.

Phasing will pick up 'NTG' patients who have a consistently low IOP. For example if a patient maintains an IOP of 14 mmHg throughout the day and they still develop glaucomatous optic neuropathy, the clinician suspects that these patients do indeed have a different disease to the higher pressure patients. These patients may behave differently and the glaucoma specialist should look for other contributory factors (see Chapter 20). A significant number of NTG patients do not progress even without treatment, so making this diagnosis does have implications for prognosis and management.

Progression despite good IOPs

In a patient who has an IOP which is apparently consistently low and yet still demonstrates evidence of progression it is important to know whether IOP-dependent damage is occurring.[10]

Patients with IOPs of 12 mmHg in the mornings may be spiking up to 18 mmHg in the afternoon. In highly compromised discs this may be enough to cause progression. There is evidence to suggest that such high fluctuation in IOP may facilitate significant damage.

Knowing the time of an IOP spike may facilitate targeted treatment, for example changing the timing of drops, or it may prompt consideration of surgical intervention. Operative intervention in the form of glaucoma surgery is known to completely flatten the diurnal curve.[11] Surgery may maintain an IOP of 12 mmHg throughout the day and thus prevent the potentially damaging diurnal rise.

Markedly varying IOP measurements

When faced with a patient who has widely ranging IOP measurements it is important to consider phasing. The time of day the IOPs have been measured will have significant implications on the IOP obtained and if these times have not been documented it will be impossible to decipher whether the different readings obtained were due to true factors (for example intermittent compliance with drops) or whether the patient's IOP is indeed varying over time.

Questionnable compliance

When faced with a patient who does not appear to respond to their medication and maintains a raised IOP sometimes it is worthwhile bringing them into a controlled environment to monitor their IOP. The patient can be visualized actually putting their drops in and a true assessment of their 'treated' IOPs can be obtained.

References

1. Armaly MF. On the distribution of applanation pressure: I. Statistical features and the effect of age, sex, and family history of glaucoma. Arch Ophthalmol 1965; 73: 11–18.
2. Vernon SA. Intraeye pressure range and pulse profiles in normals with the Pulsair Noncontact Tonometer. Eye 1993; 7: 134–137.
3. David R, Zangwill L, Briscoe D, Dagan M, Yagev R, Yassur Y. Diurnal intraocular pressure variations: an analysis of 690 diurnal curves. Br J Ophthalmol 1992; 76: 280–283.
5. Costagliola C, Trapanese A, Pagano M. Intraocular pressure in a healthy population: a survey of 751 subjects. Optom Vis Sci 1990; 67: 204–206.
4. Wilensky JT, Gieser DK, Dietsche ML, Mori MT, Zeimer R. Individual variability in the diurnal intraocular pressure curve. Ophthalmology 1993; 100: 940–944.
6. Brubaker RF. Flow of aqueous humor in humans (The Friedenwald Lecture). Invest Ophthalmol Vis Sci 1991; 32(13): 3145–3166.
7. Hasegawa K, Ishida K, Sawada A, Kawase K, Yamamoto T. Diurnal variation of intraocular pressure in suspected normal-tension glaucoma. Jpn J Ophthalmol 2006; 50: 449–454.
8. Wilensky JT, Gieser DK, Mori MT, Langenberg PW, Zeimer RC. Self-tonometry to manage patients with glaucoma and apparently controlled intraocular pressure. Arch Ophthalmol 1987; 105: 1072–1075.

9. Barkana Y, Anis S, Liebmann J, Tello C, Ritch R. Clinical utility of intraocular pressure monitoring outside of normal office hours in patients with glaucoma. Arch Ophthalmol 2006; 124: 793–797.

10. Malerbi FK, Hatanaka M, Vessani RM, Susanna R Jr. Intraocular pressure variability in patients who reached target intraocular pressure. Br J Ophthalmol 2005; 89: 540–542.

11. Konstas AG, Topouzis F, Leliopoulou O, Pappas T, Georgiadis N, Jenkins JN, Stewart WC. 24-hour intraocular pressure control with maximum medical therapy compared with surgery in patients with advanced open-angle glaucoma. Ophthalmology 2006; 113: 765.

Chapter 10

Central corneal thickness and the intraocular pressure

Why should I read this chapter?

Central corneal thickness (CCT) has become an extremely important factor in glaucoma management and particularly in consideration of ocular hypertension (OHT). There are numerous studies which indicate that corneal factors have a direct effect on the accuracy of IOP measurement. IOP reduction is a key feature of glaucoma management and therefore accurate measurement of this known risk factor is paramount. It is vital that shared care professionals have an understanding of how CCT influences IOP measurements and how to act on their readings after CCT is taken into account.

Importance of central corneal thickness

CCT is a hot topic and it is vital that the clinician understands its importance in considering treatment of glaucoma suspects or OHT patients and its effect on IOP measurements in patients who have had refractive surgery.

The importance of CCT in established glaucoma is debatable. Assuming that CCT is a constant then it should have a limited effect on patient management. When considering target IOP and whether patients achieve it, it is important to realize that CCT should have little bearing. If the patient is progressing at an IOP of 18 mmHg then they need it reducing further whether their CCT is 700 μm or 400 μm. It is potentially a factor to be taken into account when reseting the target IOP to a lower level. If the patient had a corneal thickness of 400 μm the new target IOP may be set slightly lower than the new target IOP set in the patient with a CCT of 700 μm.

It is important to separate OHT from glaucoma. It is clear that CCT is an important factor in OHT management.[1] The thinner the cornea the more likely the conversion from OHT to glaucoma (see Chapter 25).

Glaucoma management relies heavily upon IOP for the diagnosis of glaucoma but also for monitoring for progression and the response to topical, systemic or surgical treatment. When using any tool to take a clinical measurement it is important that the user understands the potential weaknesses of the technique and the potential sources of error. It is clear that CCT is a potential confounding factor in modern IOP measurement.

Goldmann applanation tonometry (GAT) remains the gold standard for IOP measurement and it should be employed methodically and routinely in every glaucoma patient. When designing the Goldmann tonometer, Goldmann and Schmidt[2] assumed that the Imbert–Fick law was valid when applied to the eye. The law states that the internal fluid pressure that acts on a thin membrane sphere is equal to the pressure that is needed to flatten a small area of that sphere. They postulated that variations in CCT occurred rarely in normal corneas and worked out all their calculations based upon a 'normal' corneal thickness of 500 µm.

Unfortunately, for several reasons, the Imbert–Fick law cannot be applied to the eye and thus the basic science behind GAT (although undeniably very clever!) is inherently flawed. Corneal biomechanics affect GAT measurements not only as a result of variations in thickness but also related to their level of individual elasticity. This does not mean that GAT is inaccurate. In the great majority of patients it still gives accurate, representative and reliable measurements of IOP.

Ehlers and colleagues[3–5] first began addressing this issue in the 1970s. Using manometry[4], they placed cannulas into the ACs of 29 normal eyes undergoing routine cataract surgery. They correlated CCT with errors in GAT measurements compared to 'true' intracameral pressure. They found that GAT most accurately reflected 'true' IOP when the CCT was 520 µm, and that deviations from this value resulted in an overestimation or underestimation of IOP by as much as 7 mmHg per 100 µm. Taken at face value this is an enormous error. Patients who we are seeing with a corneal pachymetry of 450 µm and an IOP of 21 mmHg may actually have a true IOP of 28 mmHg! *Don't panic: read on.*

One case report[6] highlighted a patient with a CCT of 900 µm with a manometric IOP of 11 mmHg, but when measured by GAT, the IOP ranged from 30–40 mmHg on maximum medical therapy. Another study[7] found that applanation tonometry underestimated IOP by as much as 4.9 mmHg in thin corneas and overestimated by up to 6.8 mmHg in thick corneas. The various studies seem to suggest a calculated correction range of 0.18–0.49 mmHg for each 10 µm change in CCT from 520 µm.

Several studies have looked at the distribution of CCT according to diagnosis in POAG, NTG and OHT. In a study by Shah *et al.*[8] normal eyes had a mean CCT of 554 µm, POAG had a mean CCT of 550 µm, NTG had a mean CCT of 514 µm and the OHT eyes had a mean CCT of 580 µm. Naturally if Ehlers[3] IOP correction criteria are applied to the above patients a significant proportion of the OHTs would be reclassified as normals, and some of the patients labelled NTG would have been reclassified as high-pressure glaucomas. One researcher[9] found that if correction factors are applied, 30% of OHT eyes could be reclassified as normal, while another group[10] found this figure to potentially be as high as 65%.

One group[11] retrospectively examined the initial visit of consecutive POAG patients over a 5-year period. They found that a lower CCT was a powerful clinical factor associated with a more marked visual-field defect, increased disc cupping, and increased number of glaucoma medications. It is possible that the initial management of the patient's glaucoma had been delayed in chronology and aggressiveness because of the reassurance of erroneously normal IOP measurements. It has been shown that a lower CCT is associated with worse baseline visual fields probably related to the aforementioned phenomenon.[12] However, in specialized hands CCT was not a useful predictor of visual field and optic disc progression. Glaucoma clinicians with an understanding of the implications of CCT on IOP measurement should not be caught out by reassuringly low IOP readings. The numbers themselves do not matter; it is the target IOP and whether the patient shows evidence of progression that matters.

In another study[13] 98 patients with pre-perimetric glaucoma (diagnosis based upon patho-logical optic discs and normal visual fields) were followed. Thirty-four patients developed a glaucomatous visual-field defect over the next 4 years. A thinner CCT predicted the develop-ment of a field defect in both univariate and multivariate analysis. Mean CCT was significantly lower in converters than in non-converters. They found that a CCT of 545 μm was the best dividing point to separate cases who developed a field defect from those who did not. At 4 years of follow-up, the cumulative probability of progressing to perimetric glaucoma was 46% in patients with a CCT less than 545 μm compared with 11% in patients with CCT over this cut off.

The Ocular Hypertension Treatment Study[14,15] has been a pivotal factor in bringing the importance of CCT to the fore of current glaucoma practice. This study has provided convinc-ing evidence that CCT is a significant risk factor for progression of OHT to POAG. This land-mark study was the first to prospectively demonstrate that a decreased CCT significantly increases the risk of developing POAG and that this was an *independent* risk factor. Participants with a CCT of 555 μm or less had a three-fold greater risk of developing POAG compared with patients who had a CCT of more than 588 μm. Measurement of CCT has an important role in the management of OHT patients.[16]

The pieces of the puzzle seemed to fall into place neatly. In theory you could measure GAT IOP and pachymetry, refer to a correction nomogram and simply read off the 'true' IOP. This would remove CCT as a confounding factor and allow us once again to concentrate on purely 'true' IOP as the risk factor for development of glaucoma.

Unfortunately the above is too good to be true as all attempts to adjust the OHTS IOP data using every published correction nomogram for GAT and CCT have failed to eliminate CCT as a predictive factor in the OHTS.

It is clear that the correction nomograms do not work for individual patients. There may be a consistent pattern or trend for patients with thicker corneas having overestimated GAT IOPs and, indeed, if 100 thick cornea patients were assessed the majority would have lower 'true' IOPs than the GAT measurements but this is far from a hard-and-fast rule. When dealing with individual patients it is dangerous to rely on correction nomograms. Because a patient has a thick CCT it does not definitely mean you are overestimating their true IOP. Generalized rules may be applied to groups of individuals (such as OHT patients as a whole) but it must be remembered that an individual patient may behave differently. You can use generalized data and evidence to treat individuals, but the clinician has to be aware that the generalized rules may not apply to the patient sitting before them.

There are two main flaws in the CCT story. CCT is only a single factor in how corneas behave.[17] Inevitably corneal collagen will behave differently between patients. Two patients with identical CCTs may have corneas which behave very differently. One may have a relatively rigid cornea and the other may have a very soft cornea, dependent upon their intrinsic amount and orientation of collagen. The patient with a rigid cornea will read an artificially higher IOP than the patient with a compliant cornea as the applanator will have to apply enough force to not only flatten against the internal IOP but also flatten the inherent rigidity of the cornea itself. This is of course a simplification and many other biological factors are inevitably at play.

The other flaw is the fact that CCT is biologically linked to other structural factors in the eye. Theoretically, the way the corneal collagen was laid down will be similar to the way the collagen of the sclera was formed. The small CCT may simply be a marker of abnormal collagen deposition throughout the eye, including at the lamina cribrosa. It is possible that the lamina cribrosa itself is structurally and dynamically different in patients with a small CCT. A previous study has found that after IOP lowering, the lamina cribrosa responded by flexing forward to a greater degree in patients with thin corneas than in those with thick corneas.[18] This movement may have pathological implications as this bouncing of the lamina cribrosa in response to a fluctuating IOP may result in pinching of optic nerve fibers as they pass through it.

There is growing evidence that the corneal rigidity (corneal hysteresis) is a more important factor than CCT *per se* in indicating how accurate our IOP readings are.

It appears that CCT is a highly heritable trait and this suggests that abnormal structural genes may be a mark of underlying glaucoma susceptibility.[19]

With the resurgence of interest in the role of CCT and corneal properties in the accuracy of IOP measurement, many new devices and technologies have been developed to try to overcome the shortcomings of GAT. Naturally there are significant financial incentives for progress in this arena: should a developer bring a proven IOP-measuring tool to the market which can replace GAT as the 'gold standard', the scope for profit is enormous.

Dynamic contour tonometry

Dynamic contour tonometry (DCT) is a relatively new device which is being marketed as being able to measure 'true' IOP independent of CCT. An electronic pressure sensor is embedded in the concave-shaped tonometer tip. Rather than applanating/flattening the cornea (and thus falling into the trap of involving corneal biomechanics) the DCT forces the central disc area of the cornea into the same shape as the tip. This theoretically allows the device to measure the true pressure of the eye because the corneal contours are matched on the inner and outer surface meaning that the pressures either side are supposedly equal.

The IOP recorded by the DCT is the mean diastolic IOP during the period the tonometer was in contact with the eye. One group of researchers[20] performed a prospective, cross-sectional observation and instrument validation study. Pachymetry, DCT, pneumatonometry and GAT were performed in a randomized order on more than 200 patients. IOP as measured by DCT, pneumatonometry and GAT were compared with each other and with CCT. They found that DCT and pneumatonometry were not significantly correlated with CCT. IOP measured by GAT, on the other hand, was dependent on CCT.

Another study[21] measured 130 eyes of 130 patients by GAT and DCT. The effect of CCT and age on GAT/DCT differences was assessed by linear regression analysis. They found that GAT was significantly more affected than DCT by both CCT and the subject's age. This suggested that in addition to CCT there was an age-related corneal biomechanical change that may be partly responsible for inducing measurement error. Other studies[22–25] have also reported that DCT is less dependent on CCT than GAT or non-contact air-puff on normal eyes and in eyes after LASIK.

One study[26] assessed GAT and DCT both pre- and post-LASIK. They found that GAT readings were on average 3.3 mmHg lower than pre-operatively but the DCT readings remained unchanged despite the surgical thinning of the CCT. Another study[27] found a similar consistency in DCT measurements after refractive surgery.

There is still no hard-and-fast evidence to suggest that the DCT does indeed measure 'true' IOP. Much more work needs to be done before this tool can be accepted and clinical decisions made upon its readings. Longer-term studies validating this in the management of glaucoma are required.

Ocular response analyzer

The ocular response analyzer (ORA) (Reichart) has been recently developed in the hope of addressing the corneal component of IOP measurement head on. It determines corneal biomechanical properties (hysteresis) using an applied force–displacement relationship and then works out IOP from these indices. A jet of air similar to that utilized in traditional air-puff tonometers generates an applanating force on the cornea. The key to this technology is the fact that two readings are taken at two different points in the applanating process. As the pressure from the air puff is applied the cornea is progressively indented becoming centrally flat and then becoming slightly concave as the pressure goes beyond the applanating cut-off. Normal air puff tonometers take this applanated point as the end-point and work out IOP from there. The ORA now gradually reduces the force of air in a curvilinear fashion. As the pressure reduces the cornea slowly bounces back to return to its normal convex nature. At a certain force it will become flat again as it goes from concave to convex. The force required to originally flatten the cornea is not the same as the force which is being applied at the time the cornea flattens on the rebound. This difference is related to the inherent biomechanical properties of the cornea and relates to hysteresis. Measurements of several populations of patients[28] indicated that corneal hysteresis varied over a large range and was only weakly correlated with CCT, perhaps explaining why simple IOP correction nomograms do not work in calculating true IOP.

There is evidence that the cornea-corrected IOPs provided by the ORA are indeed CCT independent.[29] Like DCT, there has also been a study showing that post-LASIK IOPs were unchanged when measured by the ORA, indicating potential independence from CCT.[27]

Rebound tonometry

The rebound tonometer (RBT) is a device which has not yet seen widespread clinical use. It is an assembly of two coaxial coils running down the shaft of the device that bounce a magnetized probe off the cornea and detect its deceleration caused by contact with the ocular surface. The inverse of the probe's deceleration speed is supposed to correlate with IOP.[30] The main advantage of RBT over GAT in humans is the fact that measurements can be taken without the need for topical anesthesia and with minimal discomfort.

A cross-sectional study[31] has compared measurements obtained using the RBT and GAT in 147 eyes of 85 patients with OHT or glaucoma. They found that RBT was a reproducible method of determining IOP in humans, but that it tends to overestimate IOP compared with GAT. Both tonometers were similarly affected by changes in CCT making its superiority or even equivalence to GAT questionable.

Post-LASIK eyes

The corneal bed underlying the flap becomes the load-bearing structure after LASIK.[32] The CCT measurements post-surgery cannot be used for accurate correction of IOP measurements as the biomechanical properties of the cornea would have been completely changed. Patients should be specifically asked regarding any previous history of refractive surgery, as markedly high 'true' IOPs may be missed due to apparently normal measurements in iatrogenically thinned corneas. Although correction nomograms are not reliable a high index of suspicion for underestimation of IOP should be maintained in such patients. If devices are available which are independent of CCT they should be used in these post-refractive surgery patients.[27,33]

Conclusion

The effect of CTT on GAT is not as simple as it may appear. Using generalized correction nomograms will lead to systematic errors which may have detrimental effects in some patients due to overtreatment or, of more concern, undertreatment in the setting of the reassurance of a thick cornea. The role of CCT in OHT patients is undeniable and the use of pachymetry before management decisions in these patients is essential. Use of CCT in established glaucoma is less clear. Close monitoring for signs of progression should dictate a target IOP independent of the CCT.

The biomechanics of the cornea are under the spotlight and will hopefully open avenues to new non-invasive techniques for getting a true assessment of IOP independent of corneal differences between patients.

Clinicians must take CCT into account when assessing patients who do not seem to be behaving in the way their GAT IOP readings indicate they should. Beware however that you are not underestimating true IOP in every patient with a thin cornea. Some patients can have a GAT IOP of 18 mmHg with a corneal thickness of 450 μm and yet have an ORA and DCT IOP of 14 mmHg. There are no hard-and-fast rules and all the information should be used in the context of the patient, their history, their visual fields and their clinical course.

References

1. Kass MA, Heuer DK, Higginbotham EJ, Johnson CA, Keltner JL, Miller JP, Parrish RK 2nd, Wilson MR, Gordon MO. The Ocular Hypertension Treatment Study: a randomized trial determines that topical ocular hypotensive medication delays or prevents the onset of primary open-angle glaucoma. Arch Ophthalmol 2002; 120: 701–713.
2. Goldmann H, Schmidt T. On applanation tonography. Ophthalmologica 1965; 150: 65–75.
3. Ehlers N, Bramsen T, Speriing S. Applanation tonometry and central corneal thickness. Acta Ophthalmol (Copenh) 1975; 53: 34–43.
4. Ehlers N, Hansen FK, Aasved H. Biometric correlations of corneal thickness. Acta Ophthalmol (Copenh) 1975; 53: 652–659.
5. Ehlers N, Hansen FK. Central corneal thickness in low-tension glaucoma. Acta Ophthalmol (Copenh) 1974; 52: 740–746.
6. Johnson M, Kass MA, Moses RA, *et al.* Increased corneal thickness simulating elevated intraocular pressure. Arch Ophthalmol 1978; 96: 664–665.
7. Whitacre MM, Stein RA, Hassanein K. The effect of corneal thickness on applanation tonometry. Am J Ophthalmol 1993; 115: 592–596.
8. Shah S, Chatterjee A, Mathai M, *et al.* Relationship between corneal thickness and measured intraocular pressure in a general ophthalmology clinic. Ophthalmology 1999; 106: 2154–2160.

9. Argus WA. Ocular hypertension and central corneal thickness. Ophthalmology 1995; 102: 1810–1812.

10. Herndon LW, Choudhri SA, Cox T, *et al*. Central corneal thickness in normal, glaucomatous, and ocular hypertensive eyes. Arch Ophthalmol 1997; 115: 1137–1141.

11. Herndon LW, Weizer JS, Stinnett SS. Central corneal thickness as a risk factor for advanced glaucoma damage. Arch Ophthalmol 2004; 122: 17–21.

12. Chauhan BC, Hutchison DM, LeBlanc RP, *et al*. Central corneal thickness and progression of the visual field and optic disc in glaucoma. Br J Ophthalmol 2005; 89: 1008–1012.

13. Medeiros FA, Sample PA, Zangwill LM, *et al*. Corneal thickness as a risk factor for visual field loss in patients with preperimetric glaucomatous optic neuropathy. Am J Ophthalmol 2003; 136: 805–813.

14. Brandt JD, Beiser JA, Kass MA, Gordon MO. Central corneal thickness in the Ocular Hypertension Treatment Study (OHTS). Ophthalmology 2001; 108: 1779–1788.

15. Gordon MO, Beiser JA, Brandt JD, *et al*. The ocular hypertension treatment study: baseline factors that predict the onset of primary open-angle glaucoma. Arch Ophthalmol 2002; 120: 714–720.

16. Brusini P, Tosoni C, Parisi L, Rizzi L. Ocular hypertension and corneal thickness: a long-term prospective study. Results after two years. Eur J Ophthalmol 2005; 15: 550–555.

17. Liu J, Roberts CJ. Influence of corneal biomechanical properties on intraocular pressure measurement: quantitative analysis. J Cataract Refract Surg 2005; 31: 146–155.

18. Lesk MR, Hafez AS, Descovich D. Relationship between central corneal thickness and changes of optic nerve head topography and blood flow after intraocular pressure reduction in open-angle glaucoma and ocular hypertension. Arch Ophthalmol 2006; 124: 1568–1572.

19. Toh T, Liew SH, MacKinnon JR, *et al*. Central corneal thickness is highly heritable: the twin eye studies. Invest Ophthalmol Vis Sci 2005; 46: 3718–3722.

20. Kniestedt C, Lin S, Choe J, *et at*. Clinical comparison of contour and applanation tonometry and their relationship to pachymetry. Arch Ophthalmol 2005; 123: 1532–1537.

21. Koetcha A, White ET, Shewry JM, *et al*. The relative effects of corneal thickness and age on Goldmann applanation tonometry and dynamic contour tonometry. Br J Ophthalmol 2005; 89: 1572–1575.

22. Siganos DS, Papastergiou Gl, Moedas C. Assessment of the Pascal dynamic contour tonometer in monitoring intraocular pressure in unoperated eyes and eyes after LASIK. J Cataract Refract Surg 2004; 30: 746–751.

23. Kaufmann C, Bachmann LM, Thiel MA. Intraocular pressure measurements using dynamic contour tonometry after laser in situ keratomileusis. Invest Ophthalmol Vis Sci 2003; 44: 3790–3794.

24. Kaufmann C, Bachmann LM, Thiel MA. Comparison of dynamic contour tonometry with Goldmann applanation tonometry. Invest Ophthalmol Vis Sci 2004; 45: 3118–3121.

25. Ku JY, Danesh-Meyer HV, Craig JP, Gamble GD, McGhee CN. Comparison of intraocular pressure measured by Pascal dynamic contour tonometry and Goldmann applanation tonometry. Eye 2006; 20: 191–198.

27. Pepose JS, Feigenbaum SK, Qazi MA, Sanderson JP, Roberts CJ. Changes in corneal biomechanics and intraocular pressure following LASIK using static, dynamic, and noncontact tonometry. Am J Ophthalmol 2007; 143: 39–47.

26. Duba I, Wirthlin AC. Dynamic contour tonometry for post-LASIK intraocular pressure measurements. Klin Monatsbl Augenheilkd 2004; 221: 347–350.

28. Luce DA. Determining the in vivo biomechanical properties of the cornea with an ocular response analyzer. J Cataract Refract Surg 2005; 31: 156–162.

29. Kotecha A, Elsheikh A, Roberts CR, Zhu H, Garway-Heath DF. Corneal thickness- and age-related biomechanical properties of the cornea measured with the ocular response analyzer. Invest Ophthalmol Vis Sci 2006; 47: 5337–5347.

30. Kontiola Al. A new electromechanical method for measuring intraocular pressure. Doc Ophthalmol 1997; 93: 265–276.

31. Martinez-de-ia-Casa JM, Garcia-Feijoo J, Castillo A, *et al*. Reproducibility and clinical evaluation of rebound tonometry. Invest Ophthalmol Vis Sci 2005; 46: 4578–4580.
32. Chang DH, Stulting RD: Change in intraocular pressure measurements after LASIK – The effect of the refractive correction and the lamellar flap. Ophthalmology 2005; 12: 1009–1016.
33. Kaufmann C, Bachmann LM, Thiel MA. Intraocular pressure measurements using dynamic contour tonometry after laser in situ keratomileusis. Invest Ophthalmol Vis Sci 2003; 44: 3790–3794.

Chapter 11

Evaluating the visual field

Why should I read this chapter?

The purpose of visual-field examination is to aid in the diagnosis and management of glaucoma. Visual fields assist in determining the severity of damage so that an initial target pressure can be set and the effectiveness of treatment can be determined by following the patient's fields for evidence of glaucoma progression.

This is a crucial test and is a cornerstone of glaucoma. Visual-field loss is why we manage glaucoma. For such an essential role in the management of this potentially blinding disease, it is critical that the visual-field examination be appropriate, reliable, accurate and repeatable.

Assessing visual fields

Despite the plethora of new technologies coming to the market we still rely heavily rely upon perimetry to diagnose glaucoma and monitor for any evidence of progression.

Any test in medicine should alter the course of the patient either by reassurance of normality or confirmation of abnormality. Before the visual-field test is done, the patient has a pre-test probability of having glaucoma. This pre-test probability is dependent upon several clinical characteristics, including the prevalence of glaucoma in that patient population, age, family history, IOP and the appearance of the ONH. The clinician will have an index of suspicion for glaucoma before the test is done. For example, if the patient has an IOP of 40mmHg and an asymmetrically cupped disc with a CDR in the affected eye of 0.9, then the likelihood the patient has glaucoma is high. Even if the visual field were entirely normal the patient would still probably have a diagnosis made of glaucoma and treatment commenced. Conversely if the IOPs were at the lower limit of normal and the discs were completely normal then the likelihood of glaucoma is low. Even should the field be abnormal the clinician may question whether the fields were true or artifactual. The two aforementioned cases have a high and low pre-test probability of glaucoma respectively and the visual field results have little effect on the eventual diagnosis.

Visual-field assessment becomes a highly useful tool when the diagnosis pre-test is equivocal. If the clinician is uncertain that the patient has glaucoma, for example the IOPs are only marginally raised and the disc only has a slightly suspicious area on the NRR, then we are suddenly relying heavily upon the outcome of the visual-field test. In this circumstance the visual-field examination is a powerful adjunct. Such a powerful tool can be dangerous, as, if it is misinterpreted, it can lead to significant misdiagnosis and subsequent patient morbidity. This fact emphasizes the need for the clinician to have an in-depth understanding of the test, its weaknesses and strengths, and to understand how to interpret the test appropriately. Proper patient and test selection are also paramount to allow realistic and clinically applicable interpretation.

Patient selection

There is no one-size-fits-all test with regard to visual-field assessment. Every patient should be capable of undertaking some form of test. The choice of test and the methods utilized to achieve it may have to be modified to take into consideration any visual, mental or physical limitations of the patient.

Age is not a limitation. Children and the extreme elderly may be capable of providing reliable results in automated perimetry. Physical constraints, such as the use of wheelchairs or neck problems may limit accessibility to the visual-field analyzer itself. With patience and care many of these physical limitations may be overcome and appropriate positioning achieved.

If the patient is not entirely comfortable then they should be allowed to rest periodically. Sometimes only one eye may be examined at a time to ensure an accurate result. Alternating the eye assessed first may be appropriate if the reliability indices of the second eye are always suboptimal. Some patients can only maintain their concentration for a finite amount of time. The tester (be they the clinician or a technician) should stay with the patient throughout the entire test to ensure that the patient remains alert, comfortable and well fixated.

There are many different types of perimeters available. The most frequently used in the UK is the Humphrey visual-field analyzer and the rest of this chapter will concentrate on this tool. The principles described here should apply to most other forms of static perimetry.

Test selection

Suprathreshold tests utilize bright light to test for the presence or absence of dense or even total scotomas (visual-field defects). Points of bright light are shone once at each portion of the retina under scrutiny. The patient then indicates when they can see the light by pressing some form of button. Threshold tests are much more valuable and function by detecting the precise depth of a scotoma, i.e. how much damage has been done. They present exact data as to how bright the target had to be to be visible in that part of the visual field. Therefore these tests can quantify the amount of glaucoma damage in that area.

Tests used include:

• Full Field 120 (F120). This is at best a rough screening tool looking for evidence of a gross visual-field defect. When the diagnosis of glaucoma is uncertain initially it may be a useful tool, as neurological field defects should show up nicely. It tends to favor the far nasal area with test points to try and pick up early nasal wedges. A positive test is defined by a total of 17 missed points or 8 missed points in any quadrant.

- Full Threshold 30-2. This is really the gold standard visual-field test. Unfortunately it is a long and laborious test, thereby limiting its clinical usefulness. It tests a total of 76 points in the patient's central 30° of visual field. The test points are 6° apart.
- Full Threshold 24-2. This is an identical test to the one above however it skips all the edge points of the 30-2, except the two most nasal points (to ensure it still picks up any nasal steps). The major benefit is that it cuts down test time by up to one fifth. It thus tests a total of 54 points in the patient's central 24° of vision with test points also 6° apart.
- Full Threshold 10-2. This tests the central 10° of vision, with 68 test points spaced 2° apart. This is an ideal test in advanced glaucoma. Whenever glaucoma progresses to a stage where fixation is threatened this test should be utilized. In the 24-2 and 30-2 point patterns, the four points closest to fixation are 4.2° away, meaning that the patient could lose significant central acuity before the scotoma was large enough to be picked up. The 68 points of the 10-2 test are only 2° apart, with the innermost four points only 1.4° from fixation, making it ideal for the assessment of the patients at greatest risk of visual loss (i.e. those with advanced glaucoma with field defects threatening fixation) (Fig. 11.1).

Most of the above tests can be performed with FASTPAC, Swedish Interactive Thresholding Algorithm (SITA) Standard, or SITA Fast programs:

- FASTPAC. Standard full threshold tests decrease the light intensity at each point in 4 dB increments. When the patient cannot see a point (patient's visual threshold for that point crossed) the machine reverses the light intensity by increasing it in 2 dB steps until the patient can see it again (crossing the visual threshold again). FASTPAC is an alternative strategy that uses 3 dB steps instead of 4 dB. In addition, once the patient cannot see the light the machine accepts that value and does not increase the intensity again to 'double check it' (thus crossing the threshold only once instead of twice). Test time is reduced by as much as 40% but some degree of accuracy is inevitably sacrificed, and certain scotomas may be underestimated. Neither the glaucoma hemifield test (GHT), which analyzes the field for a defect, nor glaucoma change probability (GCP) analysis, which looks for significant progression, is available when FASTPAC is used.
- SITA tests. The SITA Standard test strategy reduces test time even further. Even faster is the SITA Fast test. As with everything in life you don't get something for nothing, meaning that the accuracy of the faster tests is not quite up to the full threshold strategies. The SITA tests use clever computerized algorithms based upon a large normative database to work out the visual-field values for each point. It uses the thresholds in adjacent test points to work out a starting point for subsequent tests. If one point had an absolute scotoma then the likelihood is that the adjacent point will not be normal and thus it does not waste time by shining a dim light at that adjacent point but instead starts with a moderately bright one. The light sensitivities can be worked out with fewer 'questions' asked and thus the test time is reduced when compared with full threshold tests. The SITA Fast test does the same job but with slightly less scrutiny at each test point. It is thus faster but again it is not quite as reliable as the SITA Standard test.

Most clinicians tend to use the 24-2 programs in their glaucoma practice as they achieve a balance between utility, speed and accuracy. The 30-2 test can sometimes give a high rate of false-positive readings from the peripheral points. The best program for the initial and

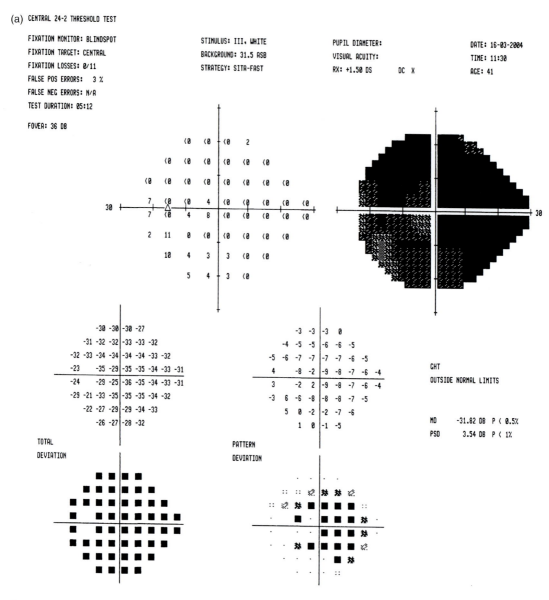

(a) CENTRAL 24-2 THRESHOLD TEST

FIXATION MONITOR: BLINDSPOT
FIXATION TARGET: CENTRAL
FIXATION LOSSES: 0/11
FALSE POS ERRORS: 3 %
FALSE NEG ERRORS: N/A
TEST DURATION: 05:12

FOVEA: 36 DB

STIMULUS: III, WHITE
BACKGROUND: 31.5 ASB
STRATEGY: SITA-FAST

PUPIL DIAMETER:
VISUAL ACUITY:
RX: +1.50 DS   DC X

DATE: 16-03-2004
TIME: 11:30
AGE: 41

GHT
OUTSIDE NORMAL LIMITS

MD   -31.82 DB P < 0.5%
PSD   3.54 DB P < 1%

TOTAL DEVIATION

PATTERN DEVIATION

Figure 11.1 Importance of 10-2. (a) 24-2 Humphreys visual field in advanced glaucoma. The whole visual field appears to be a scotoma making it useless for attempting to pick up progression. (b) 10-2 Humphreys visual field of the same patient showing the residual visual field.

(b) CENTRAL 10-2 THRESHOLD TEST

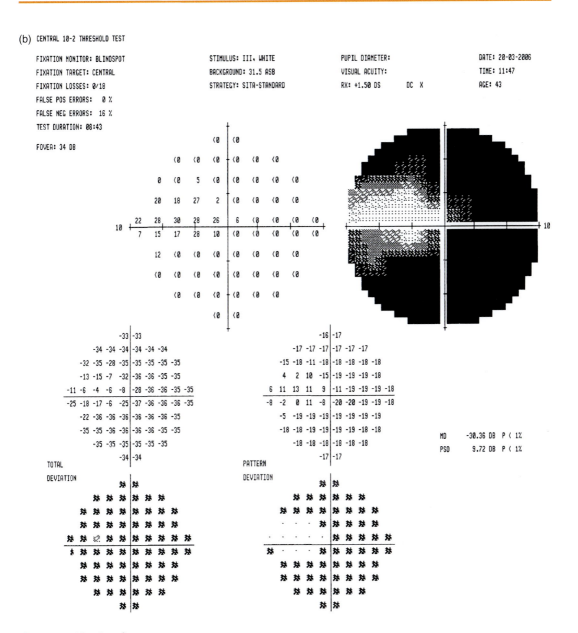

FIXATION MONITOR: BLINDSPOT STIMULUS: III, WHITE PUPIL DIAMETER: DATE: 20-03-2006

FIXATION TARGET: CENTRAL BACKGROUND: 31.5 ASB VISUAL ACUITY: TIME: 11:47

FIXATION LOSSES: 0/18 STRATEGY: SITA-STANDARD RX: +1.50 DS DC X AGE: 43

FALSE POS ERRORS: 0 %

FALSE NEG ERRORS: 16 %

TEST DURATION: 08:43

FOVEA: 34 DB

MD -30.36 DB P (1%

PSD 9.72 DB P (1%

Figure 11.1 (Continued)

subsequent visual fields is the SITA Standard 24-2. This will be suitable for the majority of patients however if the patient fatigues easily the strategy may be changed to SITA Fast. Great caution should be exercised if attempting to diagnose progression based upon visual fields taken with different test strategies. The key is to maintain consistency with regard to test conditions.

Reliability indices

Once the patient is comfortable and happy and the correct test has been chosen it is important to ensure that the test is reliable. The choice of test and the skills of the perimetrist will optimize the likelihood of a reliable outcome.

When assessing a visual field the clinician should scrutinize the reliability indices to ensure that what they are seeing is a true representation of the physiological or pathological state of the patient.

Fixation losses

The field analyzer repeatedly puts a stimulus into the patient's blind spot. If the patient can see it and responds they are clearly not fixating correctly. If there are excessive fixation losses a visual-field loss may be masked as the patient is looking around the test bowl and moving any scotoma around. The perimetrist should also observe the patient continually to give an opinion as to the patient's level of fixation and to offer encouragement to the patient if they are wavering.

False-negatives

The patient is not reacting to a stimulus placed in an area which has already proven to be seen. This may be a sign of patient fatigue but can also occur if the patient has an extensive visual-field defect. If faced with high false-negative rates it may be worthwhile changing to a faster testing strategy. The visual field may appear worse than it actually is.

False-positives

High values here indicate a 'trigger-happy' patient. They are pressing the button when no stimulus is being provided. A high false-positive rate is more worrisome than high false-negatives and can make a visual field virtually uninterpretable. Patients should have the test explained to them again and it must be emphasized that they should only press the button when they see a light.

Generally speaking false-negatives up to 20% may be acceptable while false-positives should not generally be above 10% to allow confidence in assessing the visual field.

Gaze tracking

Rather than use stimuli periodically placed in the blind spot to monitor fixation it is possible to use automatic recognition of the corneal reflexes to ensure adequate fixation.

Pseudodefects and other diseases which may mimic glaucoma

Not all visual-field defects are glaucoma and equally not all glaucoma patients with a visual-field defect have it because of their glaucoma. There are several visual-field defects that may mimic glaucoma and there are numerous apparent visual-field defects which are not really there at all.

Poor reliability or poor performance by the patient is the commonest cause of visual-field artifact. Once a patient improves on their learning curve their visual field should also improve and any false-positive visual-field defects should disappear. Most patients improve significantly over their first two or three visual-field tests. It is important to repeat the visual-field test to ensure that any defect present on the patient's first visual field is not simply learning artifact.

Improper placement of a trial lens can cause a rim artifact resulting in a concentric ring scotoma. High refractive errors (particularly high hypermetropia) can result in a significant lens rim artefact (Fig. 11.2). This effect is manifested if the patient gradually pulls back from the lens during the test.

Uncorrected refractive errors cause an overall depression right across the visual field.

Facial anatomy can have a significant effect on visual-field assessment. A large nose or excessively protruding supraorbital margins can affect visual fields. The cause of such visual-field defects should become immediately obvious when you examine the patient.

Media opacities (such as cataracts) should result in overall depression of the whole visual field. This should be corrected for automatically by the pattern standard deviation plot (see below).

Extreme pupil miosis (for example secondary to pilocarpine use) may result in apparent loss of the peripheral visual field or a generalized depression.

Defects in the upper portions of one or both eyes visual fields with a horizontal cut off may be due to ptosis. Experienced perimetrists should recognize the presence of significant lid drooping and tape the lids up.

Retinal pathology such as scars, bleeds, vaso-occlusive events, or retinal detachments will cause a field defect in the exact pattern of the affected retinal area (Fig. 7.2). Tilted discs, optic disc drusen, optic pits, anterior ischemic optic neuropathy, papillitis, chronic papilledema and toxic optic neuropathies can produce a variety of visual-field defects.

Retrochiasmal lesions (lesions of the visual pathways behind the optic chiasm) produce bilateral visual-field defects. They are homonymous (both on the same side i.e. right nasal and left temporal or right temporal and left nasal) and can be highly incongruous if anterior. This incongruity will result in a different pattern of visual-field loss in each eye which can mimic glaucoma. Neurological disease tends to obey the vertical midline but patient inconsistency or unreliability can allow these defects the appearance of crossing the vertical slightly (Fig. 11.3). It is vital to put the visual field together with the appearance of the optic nerve and other clinical parameters to avoid missing a neurological field defect (see Chapter 20).

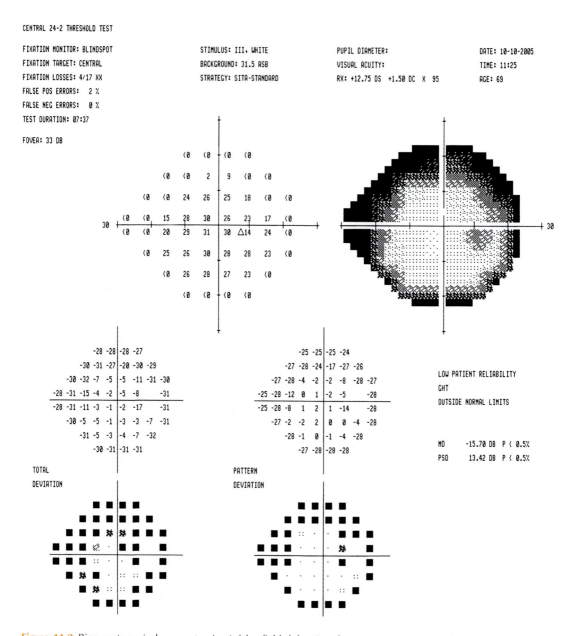

Figure 11.2 Ring scotoma in hypermetropia. A false field defect in a hypermetropic patient. The patient moves their head back during the test causing a ring defect due to edge artifact from their corrective lens.

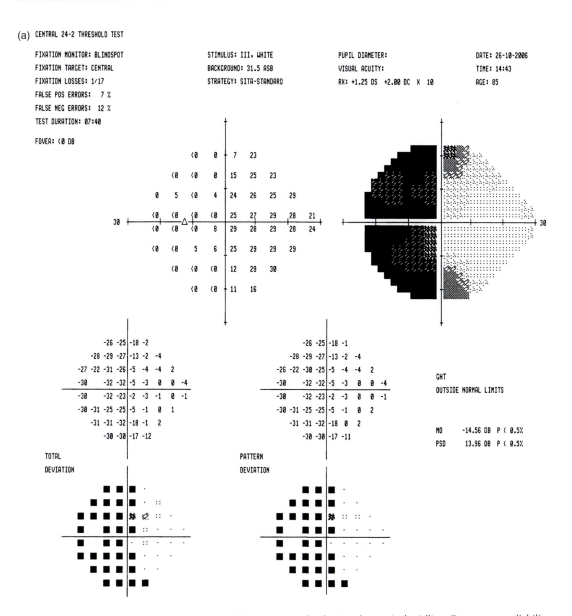

(a) CENTRAL 24-2 THRESHOLD TEST

Figure 11.3 24-2 Humphreys visual fields with defects apparently obeying the vertical midline. Due to poor reliability parts of the defect appear to cross the midline.

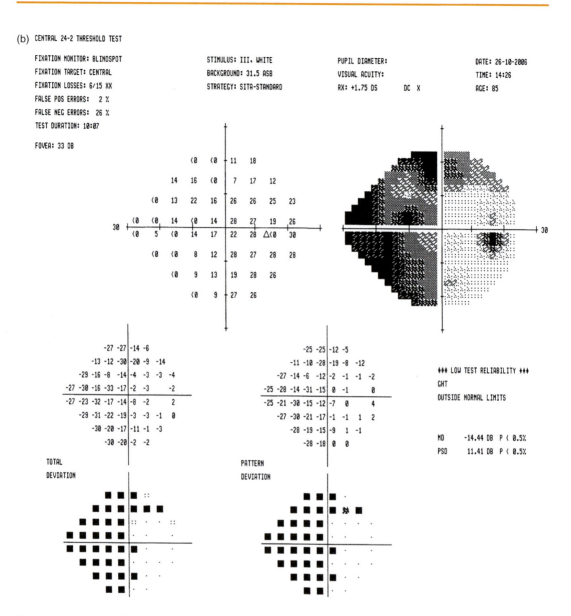

(b) CENTRAL 24-2 THRESHOLD TEST

FIXATION MONITOR: BLINDSPOT
FIXATION TARGET: CENTRAL
FIXATION LOSSES: 6/15 XX
FALSE POS ERRORS: 2 %
FALSE NEG ERRORS: 26 %
TEST DURATION: 10:07

FOVEA: 33 DB

STIMULUS: III. WHITE
BACKGROUND: 31.5 ASB
STRATEGY: SITA-STANDARD

PUPIL DIAMETER:
VISUAL ACUITY:
RX: +1.75 DS   DC X

DATE: 26-10-2006
TIME: 14:26
AGE: 85

*** LOW TEST RELIABILITY ***
GHT
OUTSIDE NORMAL LIMITS

MD   -14.44 DB P < 0.5%
PSD   11.41 DB P < 0.5%

TOTAL DEVIATION

PATTERN DEVIATION

Figure 11.3 (Continued)

Patients with unexplained bilateral visual-field defects that are greater temporally than nasally should be imaged to exclude chiasmal compression.

Visual field interpretation

Field defects commonly found in early glaucoma are:

- Nasal steps (Fig. 11.4): a nasal defect entering the visual field at the peripheral points. It tends to obey the horizontal midline and usually lies above or below this.
- Paracentral scotomas (Fig. 11.5): these defects surround fixation in various patterns. Patients with NTG may have dense scotomas quite close to fixation.
- Arcuate defects (Figs. 11.6 and 11.7): these defects lie within the retinal nerve fiber layers as they arc out of the disc and skirt the macula in a partial ellipse. This is the archetypal glaucomatous visual-field defect and may appear superiorly or inferiorly.
- Temporal wedge: a temporal visual-field defect which resembles a wedge. It usually straddles the horizontal midline.

As the disease progresses the aforementioned visual-field defects tend to coalesce eventually leaving only a temporal or central island of vision.

Interestingly clinical observation suggests that patients tend to have defects which start in one hemifield (superior or inferior) and progress only in that half of the visual field. Patients can lose a whole hemifield (effectively being left with an altitudinal defect) before they develop visual-field loss in the other hemifield. This interesting phenomenon is the basis behind the glaucoma hemifield defect (see below).

Preliminary steps:

(1) Check that the visual field belongs to the patient (it is amazing how many times the wrong visual field can end up in the clinical notes).
(2) Check that the visual field is the one you requested.
(3) Check the date – when was the field done, is it the most recent one?
(4) Check the reliability indices and decide how much notice you will take of the test – if the reliability indices are terrible you should discard the visual field completely. If the reliability is borderline then interpretation is possible but confirmatory visual-field tests should be sought before management decisions are made.

The assessment of a first visual field, i.e. the one you are making an initial diagnosis upon, is very different from follow-up visual fields. When looking at the first visual field you are asking several questions:

(1) Is this visual field normal?
(2) If not, is this glaucoma?
(3) If it is not glaucoma, is this a neurological visual-field defect or an artifact?
(4) Am I sure this is not a neurological visual-field defect?
(5) Am I really sure this is not a neurological visual-field defect?

Assessment of follow-up visual-field tests in glaucoma patients is aimed at looking for evidence of glaucoma progression (see below). In OHT patients the clinician is alert for any sign of the development of glaucoma.

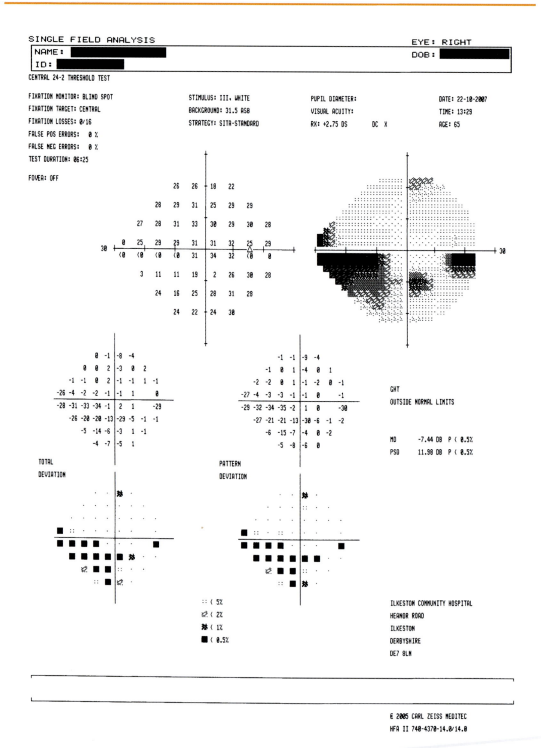

Figure 11.4 Nasal step. Humphreys 24-2 visual field showing a nasal defect which lies below the horizontal.

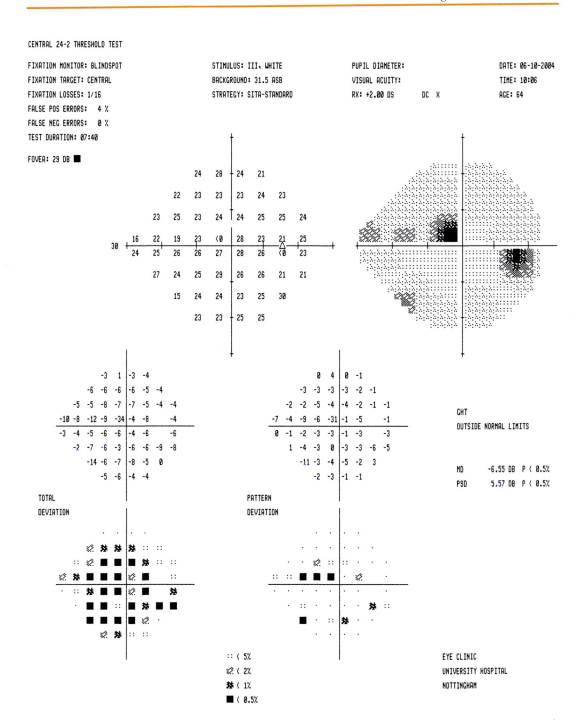

Figure 11.5 Paracentral scotoma. 24-2 Humphreys visual field showing a dense paracentral scotoma typical of normal-tension glaucoma.

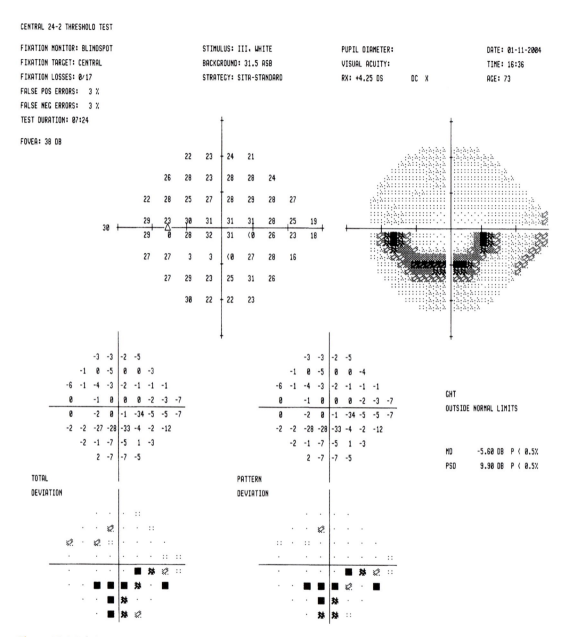

CENTRAL 24-2 THRESHOLD TEST

FIXATION MONITOR: BLINDSPOT   STIMULUS: III, WHITE   PUPIL DIAMETER: DATE: 01-11-2004
FIXATION TARGET: CENTRAL   BACKGROUND: 31.5 ASB   VISUAL ACUITY: TIME: 16:36
FIXATION LOSSES: 0/17   STRATEGY: SITA-STANDARD   RX: +4.25 DS   DC X   AGE: 73
FALSE POS ERRORS: 3 %
FALSE NEG ERRORS: 3 %
TEST DURATION: 07:24

FOVEA: 38 DB

                              22   23   24   21
                        26   28   23   28   28   24
                  22   28   25   27   28   29   28   27
            29   23   30   31   31   31   28   25   19
      30   29   0   28   32   31   (0   26   23   18
            27   27   3   3   (0   27   28   16
                  27   29   23   25   31   26
                        30   22   22   23

        -3 -3 -2 -5   -3 -3 -2 -5
     -1   0 -5   0   0 -3   -1   0 -5   0   0 -4
  -6 -1 -4 -3 -2 -1 -1 -1   -6 -1 -4 -3 -2 -1 -1 -1
     0   -1   0   0   0 -2 -3 -7   0   -1   0   0   0 -2 -3 -7   GHT
     0   -2   0 -1 -34 -5 -5 -7   0   -2   0 -1 -34 -5 -5 -7   OUTSIDE NORMAL LIMITS
  -2 -2 -27 -28 -33 -4 -2 -12   -2 -2 -28 -28 -33 -4 -2 -12
     -2 -1 -7 -5   1 -3   -2 -1 -7 -5   1 -3
        2 -7 -7 -5   2 -7 -7 -5   MD   -5.60 DB P < 0.5%
                                                                                        PSD   9.90 DB P < 0.5%
   TOTAL   PATTERN
   DEVIATION   DEVIATION

Figure 11.6 Inferior arcuate scotoma. 24-2 Humphreys visual field showing a localized inferior arcuate scotoma.

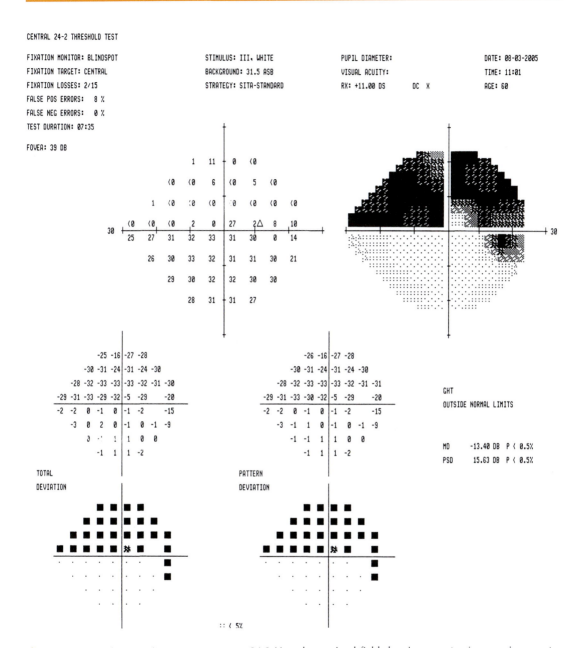

CENTRAL 24-2 THRESHOLD TEST

FIXATION MONITOR: BLINDSPOT

FIXATION TARGET: CENTRAL

FIXATION LOSSES: 2/15

FALSE POS ERRORS: 8 %

FALSE NEG ERRORS: 0 %

TEST DURATION: 07:35

FOVEA: 39 DB

STIMULUS: III, WHITE

BACKGROUND: 31.5 ASB

STRATEGY: SITA-STANDARD

PUPIL DIAMETER:

VISUAL ACUITY:

RX: +11.00 DS   DC X

DATE: 08-03-2005

TIME: 11:01

AGE: 60

TOTAL
DEVIATION

PATTERN
DEVIATION

GHT
OUTSIDE NORMAL LIMITS

MD   -13.40 DB P < 0.5%

PSD   15.63 DB P < 0.5%

:: < 5%

Figure 11.7 Extensive superior arcuate scotoma. 24-2 Humphreys visual field showing an extensive superior arcuate scotoma.

The visual field is often described as a hill of vision with increasing sensitivity to lower light stimuli as fixation is approached. This makes anatomical sense as the density of photoreceptors progressively increases towards the centre of vision. There are large normative databases for visual-field sensitivity which are incorporated into the software which analyzes the visual-field results and presents the data in the print-out.

The median value for each point in the visual field is known and moreover the normal range of values for each point is stored. We know that the closer you get to fixation the smaller the acceptable range for visual-field sensitivity. Close to fixation a patient with a sensitivity more than 5 dB less than the median may be flagged as markedly abnormal, whereas this variation from the normal value may be 'within normal limits' at a point 15° from fixation.

Humphreys 24-2 normal print-out

An example is shown in Fig. 11.8.

Grayscale plot (top right)

The grayscale print-out is helpful in examining the gross shape of a visual-field defect. It may allow a rapid impression of whether the visual-field defect fits with any of the classical patterns of glaucomatous visual-field defects or whether it may be a manifestation of a neurological or artifactual defect. The other function of the grayscale is its use in engaging the patient in their own glaucoma care. By showing the patient the plot and pointing out the 'black bits' representing their glaucoma damage they may get a true impression of the significance of their disease. Emphasizing that the 'black bit' is encroaching almost on their central vision can be a good motivator for compliance. Except for the two above reasons interpretation of the grayscale plot is of limited value.

Threshold values plot (top left)

These are the actual threshold values obtained for each point tested and are of limited clinical use. Usually, the probability plots are more useful than the actual threshold values, however the actual values can be helpful in demonstrating the raw data utilized for the other plots displayed below.

Probability values (two lower plots)

Focal sensitivity starts at a normal level in glaucoma and gradually deteriorates as the damage worsens. The probability plots compare sensitivity at each tested point with the normal database and present a visual symbol representing any deviation from this normality (i.e. outside the normal range for that age-matched point).

When the threshold value detected out of the 95th centile it is displayed as a slightly checkered square indicating a p-value of less than 5%. This means that less than 5% of the normal

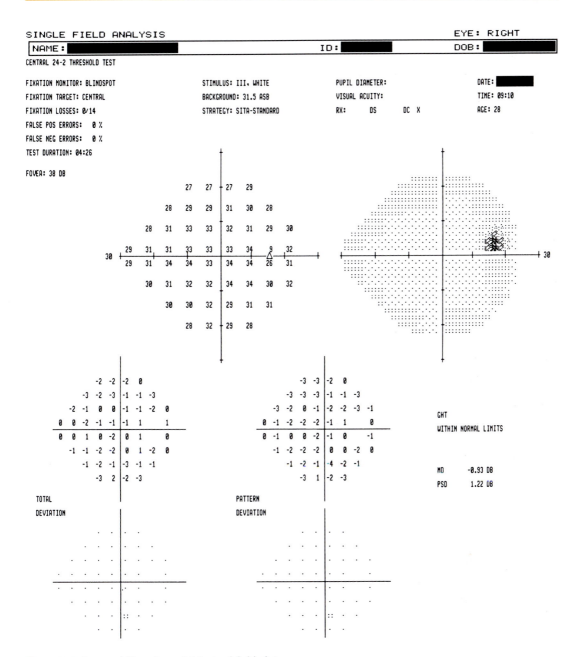

Figure 11.8 A normal Humphreys 24-2 visual field plot.

age-matched population would have a similar reading. Probability values of less than 2%, less than 1% and less than 0.5% are represented by checkers of increasing density until a black square is placed on the plot. A simple dot indicates normality for that point.

As with every statistical assessment it should be remembered that statistics are not infallible. A point with a probability point less than 2% still means that 2 out of 100 normal individuals would have a similar threshold value. In clinical practice the darker the square the greater the certainty of abnormality.

Total deviation plots (bottom left)

This plot looks at the threshold values obtained and compares them numerically (upper plot) and statistically (lower plot) to the age-matched control normative database. The numerical values portray the amount of deviation from normal. A positive value indicates that the patient is seeing better at that point that the control population would. A negative value (the sort we're unfortunately used to seeing) indicates that the patient's retinal sensitivity at that point is below normal. For example, a value of −6 indicates that the patient's threshold for that point is 6 dB below the normal (median) value. This may or may not be deemed abnormal depending on its centrality.

The retinal sensitivity is affected by any media opacities such as cataracts. A diffuse cataract will scatter the light entering the eye to some degree and cause decreased sensitivity at all retinal points tested. The software is aware of this and takes it into account by looking at all the data points and working out that some form of media opacity may be responsible for part of the global decreased sensitivity seen. If all the points are more than 5 dB below normal the analysis may surmise that this diffuse loss is probably due to some form of media opacity. The software recalculates all the data points by incorporating this 'fiddle factor' and produces a pattern deviation plot.

It is important to recognize that this may or may not be an appropriate correction. When faced with a large difference between the total deviation plot and the pattern deviation plot it is important that the clinician confirms that a media opacity is indeed present. Sometimes glaucoma itself can cause a generalized loss of sensitivity, a fact which would be completely missed by the corrective sensitivity upgrading of the pattern deviation data.

Pattern deviation plots (bottom right)

When a new value for each tested point has been calculated, it is displayed as a numerical factor (upper plot) and also compared with the normal database, once more giving a statistical plot (lower plot). When no significant diffuse loss in sensitivity is seen, the total and pattern deviation plots are identical. These plots are generally considered to be the most valuable in the setting of glaucoma management.

In a patient with advanced glaucoma and only a small central island of vision remaining the total deviation values at nearly all the points may be so depressed that the software assumes that there must be massive media opacity. It corrects all the abnormal points up to normality and moves the few remaining central normal points up to supranormal values. This makes the pattern deviation plot white in the peripheries and black in the centre (because the supranormal values are abnormally high in sensitivity) and is called pattern deviation reversal (Fig. 11.9).

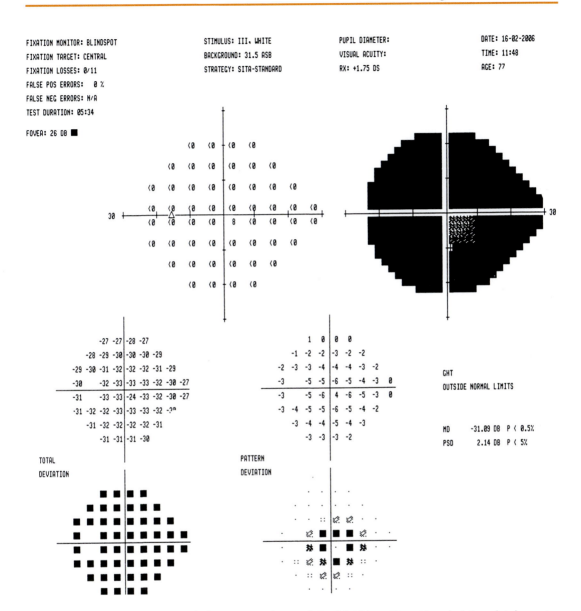

FIXATION MONITOR: BLINDSPOT
FIXATION TARGET: CENTRAL
FIXATION LOSSES: 0/11
FALSE POS ERRORS: 0 %
FALSE NEG ERRORS: N/A
TEST DURATION: 05:34

FOVEA: 26 DB ■

STIMULUS: III, WHITE
BACKGROUND: 31.5 ASB
STRATEGY: SITA-STANDARD

PUPIL DIAMETER:
VISUAL ACUITY:
RX: +1.75 DS

DATE: 16-02-2006
TIME: 11:48
AGE: 77

GHT
OUTSIDE NORMAL LIMITS

MD   -31.09 DB P < 0.5%
PSD   2.14 DB P < 5%

TOTAL
DEVIATION

PATTERN
DEVIATION

Figure 11.9 Pattern deviation reversal plot. A severe degree of visual-field loss. The pattern deviation plot shows statistical abnormality centrally due to supposed hypersensitivity. This is an artifact due to the erroneous upward correction of all the sensitivity points.

Global indices

The global indices are helpful for generalized assessment of the status of the visual field at any one point in time. The values computed are weighted to give more emphasis on the points closer to fixation. Thus peripheral defects tend to affect these indices to a much lesser degree than any defects occurring in the paracentral region. A statistical analysis is provided next to these indices comparing them to the age-matched normal population. A value less than 0.5% indicates a likelihood of significant global abnormality.

In order to address global loss of visual field sensitivity and focal loss two indices are provided, the mean deviation and the pattern standard deviation.

Mean deviation

The mean deviation (MD) is the average difference of each point from its statistically expected value. It gives a quick assessment of the overall condition of the patient's whole field. In advanced glaucoma it can help in the detection of progression as it will deteriorate progressively as the glaucoma worsens. It is not a useful tool when trying to detect glaucoma as small early defects are lost completely because they are averaged out with the rest of the normal field. It is also prone to being influenced by media opacities.

Pattern standard deviation

The pattern standard deviation (PSD) picks up any local areas of reduced field sensitivity. It measures the smoothness of the 'hill of vision' and is abnormal when there are significant depressions in that hill. Next to the numeric value is a computed probability value, which only appears when it falls outside of the 95% range of normalilty.

Summary

In assessing a visual-field test you:

(1) Look at the grayscale image and decide whether it is a neurological pattern of field defect. If there is a defect you might show it to the patient to engage them in their disease. You then ignore the grayscale and move on to the formal assessment of the visual field.
(2) Now you look at the total deviation and pattern deviation plots to see whether any areas of statistically reduced sensitivity are highlighted. If there is a significant difference between the total deviation and pattern deviation plots you need to assess clinically whether the patient has media opacity to account for this difference. If there is media opacity then the pattern deviation plot is the one you need to concentrate on. If there is no such media opacity the total deviation plot may be the true representation of the patient's visual field.
(3) Look at the statistical plots but go beyond the black squares. Look at the actual sensitivity comparisons, i.e. look at each point and see how far from normality it is deviated. A black square could indicate a −10 dB defect or a −30 dB defect. These are of course representative

of a very different degree of glaucomatous damage and, more importantly, functional damage. Of vital relevance is that a patient could progress from a point field defect of −10 dB to −30 dB with no change in that aforementioned black square. Compare each point to the values obtained on previous fields to try and detect progression (see below).

(4) Now look at the global indices to see what the MD and PSD show. Compare them to previously obtained values.
(5) Decide now whether this field is glaucomatous or not.
(6) *Whatever you decide, does it fit with the clinical picture?*
(7) Consider repeating the visual-field test again if the clinical situation allows, confirming or refuting your findings. Often several repeated visual fields are required before any definitive statements can be made.

Diagnosing glaucoma from the visual field

You cannot diagnose glaucoma from a visual field alone. You can have a field defect which is consistent with glaucomatous optic neuropathy but the diagnosis is a completely different issue which relies upon the other clinical features of the patient. It is essential that the visual-field defect fits with the optic disc. If you see a defect which appears to be an early inferior arcuate then the diagnosis may or may not be glaucoma. If the patient also has a notch in the superior disc rim and a pressure of 45 mmHg then the visual field is probably consistent with glaucoma. Conversely, if the disc is completely normal and the IOP is 12 mmHg then the likelihood is that the defect is an artifact. In the former case the patient clearly needs treatment whereas in the latter case there is plenty of room for maneuver. The patient will not be harmed by taking the time to repeat the visual-field test.

Normal patients do not always have normal visual fields. Single abnormal points are not uncommon. These may appear as black squares on the pattern deviation plot indicating severe abnormality but they may actually be complete artifact and disappear on repeat testing. It is important to look at the precise figures on the numeric plot to determine exactly how abnormal that point is.

Whenever assessing a visual-field print-out it is important to remember the pathogenesis of the visual-field defect, i.e. glaucoma. Glaucoma is unlikely to markedly affect only one part of the retina but leave the adjacent areas completely intact. However localized an optic disc notch is it will result in damage to a significant number of retinal nerve fibers. Losing only one point of the visual field is unlikely. Glaucoma usually manifests as clusters of defects on the visual field. There may be one focus which is more damaged than the adjacent ones but those adjacent areas are usually subnormal even though they may not dip into marked statistical significance. Looking at the numbers rather than the probability plot will allow the clinician to determine which clusters are of greater suspicion. Usually three or more contiguous points on the same side of the horizontal meridian are deemed to be of concern. When the whole visual field is depressed by media opacity or miosis the occurrence of artifactual clusters may increase. This should however be fully corrected for in the pattern deviation plot.

The glaucoma hemifield test

This test relies on the fact that one hemifield tends to be damaged first in glaucoma, relatively sparing the other half. Therefore, one hemifield can be used as the control and comparison made with the other half, i.e. superior compared with inferior or vice versa. The clinician can do this manually by comparing mirror image points above and below the horizontal midline, but this is time consuming.

Asman and Heiji formalized this cross-meridional strategy by developing the GHT.[1,2] This uses different paired sectors above and below the horizontal to theoretically target the areas of commonest RNFL loss. By statistically comparing the sensitivity readings of these areas the analysis can provide information as to whether the results are 'outside normal limits', 'borderline' or 'within normal limits'.

The GHT analysis is done automatically and displayed on the print-out. As with every tool it does not replace the need for methodical scrutiny of the visual field by the clinician as described above. The GHT results are defined as below:

- Outside normal limits: either an upper zone differs from its corresponding lower zone at a p < 1% level, or two corresponding zones are both depressed relative to normal at a p < 0.5% level.
- Borderline: an upper zone differs from its corresponding lower zone at a p < 3% level, but above the p < 1% level.
- General reduction sensitivity: the overall height of the hill of vision is reduced at a p < 0.5% level, but the field does not satisfy the criteria for outside normal limits. The field may be borderline.
- Within normal limits: none of the above criteria is met.

The clinician makes the diagnosis and is responsible for methodical, systematic and thorough scrutiny of the visual-field results. Once the results are noted the interpretation begins. Interpretation cannot and must not be carried out in isolation. All the clinical features should be taken into account as well as the results of all previous sequential fields before any judgment is made.

Classifying the severity of field loss

Methods to classify the degree of visual-field loss can occupy pages of text. There are numerous algorithms available to stratify the stage of glaucoma damage based on visual fields. Whether a firm classification of the visual-field loss is necessary in day-to-day clinical practice is debatable.

The degree of visual-field loss and its pattern are certainly important as they have a direct bearing upon the patient and their likely prognosis. Moreover severity will play an important part in setting an initial target IOP (see Chapter 15).

The clinician will rapidly get used to classifying visual fields according to intuitive criteria. If a patient has only slight evidence of an arcuate scotoma with only two or three points involved then their field defect is mild. If they only have a central island of vision left, their field loss is very severe. Moderate and severe defects lie somewhere in between. Making the definition between two categories does not benefit the patient directly. Generally speaking the MD is a good tool to stratify degree of field loss; less than −6 dB loss may be deemed to be mild, −6 dB to −12 dB a moderate field defect, more than −12 dB a severe visual-field defect and, finally, a defect more than −24 dB very severe loss. Again a warning has to be issued to take the whole clinical picture into account, as reliance on MD alone may falsely reassure the clinician. A defect close to fixation (as commonly seen in NTG) is of much more clinical significance and concern than an equally deep defect in the nasal periphery.

References

1. Asman P, Heiji A. Glaucoma hemifield test. Automated visual field evaluation. Arch Ophthalmol 1992; 110: 812–819.
2. Asman P, Heiji A. Evaluation of methods for automated hemifield analysis in perimetry. Arch Ophthalmol 1992; 10: 820–826.

Chapter 12

Other perimetry devices

Why should I read this chapter?

Although we have concentrated so far on standard automated perimetry there are other devices which use different technologies to detect the presence or absence of field defects. It is important that the glaucoma clinician understands their strengths and weaknesses and knows how to interpret the findings appropriately.

Short wavelength automated perimetry

Short wavelength automated perimetry (SWAP) was developed in the mid 1990s in the hope of providing a more sensitive method of assessing visual fields. Many patients with early glaucomatous optic neuropathy fail to show visual-field loss on conventional white-on-white perimetry (such as the Humphrey visual-field analyzer). This has been described as pre-perimetric glaucoma; there is evidence, however, that these patients may exhibit defects on other forms of perimetric tests such as the SWAP.

SWAP uses a large blue stimulus against a bright yellow background instead of a bright white stimulus on a background of diffuse whiteness. Several clinical studies have shown that SWAP can identify a visual-field defect before it is detected by white-on-white perimetry, and that SWAP can detect progression of the defect before it is found with standard perimetry.[1-4] Visual-field defects detected by SWAP may precede white-on-white defects by 5 or even 10 years, making it a promising tool for early detection of glaucoma.[5]

There are two main theories which aim to explain SWAP's sensitivity. It is possible that the blue light pathways are preferentially damaged in glaucoma or that these pathways have less redundancy. Because there are fewer axons in the normal eye that respond to the blue light stimulus, any diffuse loss caused by glaucoma may theoretically preferentially affect this smaller subsystem.[6,7]

Although SWAP may be more sensitive in detecting defects, it may have significant drawbacks with regard to specificity. SWAP perimetry displays greater short-term fluctuation and long-term fluctuation than does standard white-on-white perimetry,[8] making detection of progression troublesome. Media opacities such as cataracts may also result in significant artifact defects.[9]

In a study of 38 OHT patients and 62 age-matched normal control subjects, Johnson and coworkers found that both eyes of all of the OHT patients (76 eyes of 38 patients) had normal white-on-white automated perimetry but that nine of these eyes had abnormal SWAP results. Five years later, five of the nine OHT eyes with initial SWAP abnormalities had developed field defects by white-on-white perimetry as well. In contrast, none of the 67 OHT eyes with initially normal SWAP results developed abnormal white-on-white results during the follow-up period. Furthermore, white-on-white abnormalities that developed in the initially abnormal SWAP-tested eyes occurred in the same region of the visual field that was abnormal on short wavelength testing. The authors thus concluded that SWAP defects can precede glaucomatous field loss detected by standard white-on-white perimetry.[10]

In a later study, Demirel and Johnson examined 500 eyes of 250 patients with OHT and compared these visual-field results to normative data derived from examinations of 60 normal subjects. Baseline prevalence of SWAP defects was 9.4% in the patients with OHT and 1.4% in the normal population. During the study the rates of field loss were approximately 1.2% per year for both SWAP and standard automated perimetry.[11] The similar incidence rates suggested both measures are detecting the same disease process, i.e. glaucoma progression. The higher initial prevalence rate supports the belief that SWAP is more sensitive to early glaucomatous defects than white-on-white perimetry.

Despite promising features there are significant problems with SWAP technology. SWAP testing tends to take a significantly longer time than white-on-white perimetry, making it relatively patient unfriendly. It also has a significant learning effect.[12] In addition because of the reduced redundancy of the axons which serve detection of blue light stimuli (the feature which makes the SWAP good for early glaucoma) patients with moderate to severe white-on-white field loss show a much worse visual field as they have already lost most of their blue sensitive axons.[13] This makes SWAP unsuitable for patients with moderate to advanced glaucoma.

At present SWAP is not recommended as a substitute for standard white-on-white perimetry. It may have a role in patients who have morphological features to suggest glaucoma (such as NRR loss or RNFL defects) but have normal visual fields, i.e. pre-perimetric glaucoma. Detecting a visual-field defect in this situation may help in prevention of early progression and tailoring therapy to stop the patient breaching the threshold into white-on-white defects.

Frequency-doubling technology perimetry

Another new perimetry device which aims to beat conventional white-on-white testing is frequency-doubling technology (FDT). The frequency-doubling perimeter (FDP) is a compact and portable unit that does not require any special testing area.

In the standard central 20° test, stimuli are presented at 17 locations: one central 5° target and four 10° peripheral targets per quadrant. The stimulus used in FDP is a grating of very low spatial frequency (narrow width) that is flickered at a high temporal frequency (25 flickers per second). The light and dark bars alternate 25 times a second. At the right combination of spatial and temporal frequencies the total number of bars appears to double. During the test, the contrast of the stimulus is varied, and the patient is asked to respond when they notice a dark, flickering stimulus.

Frequency doubling is a phenomenon mediated by the neural pathways necessary for detecting motion (the magnocellular pathway).[14] The magnocellular pathway is comprised of large-diameter axons that make up only 15% of the total number of axons in the normal eye. Of these about a third are connected to M-cells which are responsible for the frequency doubling phenomenon. These M-cells are thought to be preferentially affected in early glaucoma. In addition because they have so little redundancy (i.e. there are so few of them that any losses will have a significant effect), it is thought that testing of this specific pathway will pick up defects earlier than standard perimetry.

Early research appears reasonably encouraging.[15–18] This device probably has a role in screening for glaucoma as a result of its excellent sensitivity and specificity and the fact that in the screening mode the test takes less than 1 minute per eye.

The FDP provides two levels of screening test on a large database. The screening tests evaluate the central 20° of the visual field and allow the clinician to choose either the C20-5 or C20-1 versions:

- C20-5 screening test: a stimulus known to be seen by 95% of normals is presented. If this stimulus is not seen it presents a stimulus seen by 98% of normals, and finally if this is not seen a stimulus usually seen by 99% of normals is presented.
- C20-1 screening test: a stimulus known to be seen by 99% of normals is presented first. If this stimulus is not seen it presents a stimulus seen by 99.5% of normals. If that stimulus is also not seen, the instrument presents a stimulus of maximum contrast.

Severe defects are identified when no stimuli are seen at a particular point. Any patient failing either the C20-1 or C20-5 screening requires standard white-on-white perimetry.

The screening programs of the FDP test only the central 20° and may thus miss more peripheral nasal steps which may be picked up on H24-2 or H30-2 testing. Small scotomas may be missed with FDP as the test target is larger than that used in standard perimetry. One of the major plus points is the fact that testing time is much shorter, which may mean reduced fatigue-induced artifact.

At present this technology is in development and its precise role in glaucoma is unclear. It probably has a role as a screening tool mainly due to its short test time and good sensitivity. It currently has no role in glaucoma follow-up and thus cannot be used exclusively for glaucoma management.

Summary

It appears that SWAP can detect visual-field loss earlier than standard threshold automated perimetry. However it is a lengthy, and demanding test, and is sensitive to media opacities. It has a greater magnitude of long-term fluctuation compared with standard threshold automated perimetry, making it difficult to assess disease progression accurately. FDT perimetry has a short testing time and is resistant to blur and pupil size; it may be a useful screening tool.

Further work is required before definitive recommendations are made with regards the use of these devices. They currently cannot replace standard white-on-white perimetry for glaucoma management.

References

1. Teesalu P, Airaksinen PJ, Tuulonen A. Blue-on-yellow visual field and retinal nerve fiber layer in ocular hypertension and glaucoma. Ophthalmology 1998; 105: 2077–2081.
2. Demirel S, Johnson CA. Incidence and prevalence of short wavelength automated perimetry deficits in ocular hypertensive patients. Am J Ophthalmol 2001; 131: 709–715.

3. Johnson CA, Adams AJ, Casson EJ, *et al*. Blue on yellow perimetry can predict the development of glaucomatous visual field loss. Arch Ophthalmol 1993; 111: 645–650.

4. Johnson CA, Adams AJ, Casson EJ, *et al*. Progression of early glaucomatous visual field loss as detected by blue-on-yellow perimetry and standard white-on-white automated perimetry. Arch Ophthalmol 1993; 111: 651–656.

5. Sit AJ, Medeiros FA, Weinreb RN. Short-wavelength automated perimetry can predict glaucomatous standard visual field loss by ten years. Semin Ophthalmol 2004; 19: 122–124.

6. Lynch S, Demirel S, Johnson C. Are early losses of visual function in glaucoma selective or non-selective? Invest Ophthalmol Vis Sci 1996; 34: S410.

7. Johnson CA. Selective versus nonselective losses in glaucoma. J Glaucoma 1994; 3(suppl): S32–S44.

8. Wild JM, Moss ID, Whitaker D, O'Neill EC. The statistical interpretation of blue-on-yellow visual field loss. Invest Ophthalmol Vis Sci 1995; 36: 1398–1410.

9. Moss ID, Wild JM, Whitaker DJ. The influence of age-related cataract on blue on yellow perimetry. Invest Ophthalmol Vis Sci 1995; 36: 764–773.

10. Demirel S, Johnson CA. Isolation of short-wavelength sensitive mechanisms in normal and glaucomatous visual field regions. J Glaucoma 2000; 9: 63–73.

11. Demirel S, Johnson CA. Incidence and prevalence of short wavelength automated perimetry deficits in ocular hypertensive patients. Am J Ophthalmol 2001; 131: 709–715.

12. Rossetti L, Fogagnolo P, Miglior S, Centofanti M, Vetrugno M, Orzalesi N. Learning effect of short-wavelength automated perimetry in patients with ocular hypertension. J Glaucoma 2006; 15: 399–404.

13. Johnson CA, Adams AJ, Casson EJ, *et al*. Progression of early glaucomatous visual field loss as detected by blue-on-yellow perimetry and standard white-on-white automated perimetry. Arch Ophthalmol 1993; 111: 651–656.

14. Maddess T, Henry GH. Performance of nonlinear visual units in ocular hypertension and glaucoma. Clin Vis Sci 1992; 7: 371–383.

15. Johnson CA, Samuels SJ. Screening for glaucomatous visual field loss with frequency doubling perimetry. Invest Ophthalmol Vis Sci 1997; 38: 413–425.

16. Quigley HA. Identification of glaucomatous visual field abnormality with the screening protocol of frequency doubling perimetry. Am J Ophthalmol 1998; 6: 819–829.

17. Leeprechanon N, Giangiacomo A, Fontana H, *et al*. Frequency-doubling perimetry: comparison with standard automated perimetry to detect glaucoma. Am J Ophthalmol 2007; 143: 263–271.

18. Landers JA, Goldberg I, Graham SL. Detection of early visual field loss in glaucoma using frequency-doubling perimetry and short-wavelength automated perimetry. Arch Ophthalmol 2003; 121: 1705–1710.

Section 2

Detecting progression

One of the key considerations in glaucoma management is the detection of progression. Early detection of worsening of glaucomatous optic neuropathy should allow rapid intervention in order to arrest deterioration and prevent irreversible worsening of visual field loss. Identifying glaucoma progression is a significant challenge and an accurate and reliable method of definitive detection is one of the holy grails of modern glaucoma practice.

Glaucoma progression may manifest as either structural changes in either optic nerve head appearance or retinal nerve fiber layer profile or as functional changes in the form of visual-field loss. It may be argued that the latter is the more important as we are treating the patient to prevent morbidity, and preservation of their visual function is of paramount importance to us as clinicians. There is, however, evidence to suggest that structural changes manifest before functional visual-field loss subsequently ensues. It is unknown whether intervention at the stage of morphological deterioration will prevent visual-field loss or have any benefit on visual quality-of-life indices.

It is generally accepted (and seems to make clinical sense) that the earlier progression is detected, the greater the likelihood is that expeditious treatment will prevent vision loss.

For patients with elevated IOP, significantly predictive factors for eventual progression are older age, advanced perimetric damage, smaller neuroretinal rim, large IOP fluctuations and larger area of beta-zone of parapapillary atrophy.[1,2]

References

1. Nouri-Mahdavi K, Hoffman D, Coleman AL, Liu G, Li G, Gaasterland D, Caprioli J. Advanced Glaucoma Intervention Study. Predictive factors for glaucomatous visual field progression in the Advanced Glaucoma Intervention Study. Ophthalmology 2004; 111: 1627–1635.
2. Martus P, Stroux A, Budde WM, Mardin CY, Korth M, Jonas JB. Predictive factors for progressive optic nerve damage in various types of chronic open-angle glaucoma. Am J Ophthalmol 2005; 139: 999–1009.

Chapter 13

Identifying progressive visual-field loss

Why should I read this chapter?

Detecting progression early is vital. However low we get the IOP we still worry about progression of glaucoma. Unchecked it is the progression which blinds our patients and it is progression which is our enemy. If we detect it early we can intervene (usually in the form of lowering IOP further) to stop it in its tracks and spare our patients. Identifying progression is surprisingly difficult and the question 'is the visual field getting worse?' is often not easily or confidently answered. This chapter will help you in this task.

Visual fields tend to be static however visual-field tests are unfortunately far from static. The same patient doing a visual-field test on consecutive days will show some degree of variation in their results. This variation will increase significantly when the time between examinations is increased, even if the patient's condition is actually unchanged. In the early stages of management there will be a learning effect as the patient gets used to the test and the testing conditions. Anxiety will decrease and visual-field test reliability should progressively improve. Unfortunately the patient is also aging and ocular and systemic comorbidities may be building up to make the process of visual-field testing progressively harder. Even when the patient has reached the plateau on their learning curve there is still some element of dynamic physiological variation in the results obtained. This phenomenon is termed the long-term visual-field fluctuation and is the thorn in the side of the clinician attempting to detect glaucoma progression early.

Visual-field fluctuation

In order to identify visual-field progression secondary to suboptimally controlled glaucoma, the clinician must pin-point changes that exceed the level of the patient's individual and unique long-term fluctuation (LTF). In addition to detecting a change the clinician has to be certain that the change is consistent with glaucoma and correlate this defect with other signs of progression, for example changes in NRR or RNFL.

The degree of inter-test variability (long-term fluctuation (LTF)) varies from patient to patient and, to make life harder, it tends to be more pronounced in patients with more advanced field loss. The only way to determine the LTF/noise of a patient's visual field is with serial assessments. By examining a succession of previous visual fields a judgment can be made of how much a patient's visual field can worsen only to bounce back to baseline again. It is prudent to obtain one or more confirmatory visual-field tests before apparent deterioration or development of a new visual-field defect is accepted as a marker for advancing glaucoma (Fig. 13.1). Again the number of confirmatory visual-field tests required will vary according to the clinical scenario. When faced with a patient who appears to have had a marked progression of their superior arcuate *and* clinical assessment reveals clear progression of their inferior NRR loss and an IOP of 28 mmHg, the need for confirmatory testing is equivocal. In this scenario if everything fits with progression then the patient has probably progressed. When the situation is not so clear cut there is usually sufficient time to arrange confirmatory (or hopefully refuting) visual-field tests.

Several studies have determined that in stable glaucoma patients, the deeper the initial defect, the greater the fluctuation between tests.[1-4] Therefore, the more extensive the initial field loss, the more the visual field fluctuates, even in stable glaucoma patients. Clearly it is vital to pick up progression early in patients who have advanced field loss as they have less residual visual field 'to play with' and yet (infuriatingly!) it is these patients who have the greatest LTF or visual field 'noise'. Picking progression out from this background noise is taxing, particularly as the stakes are relatively higher for these individuals.

At present, there is no widely accepted standard for defining visual-field progression and certainly none that is easily clinically applicable. Numerous clever and detailed algorithms have been created for clinical trials to define it in a standardized and scientific manner. The lack of consensus regarding the precise definition of visual-field progression is highlighted by the fact that each of the recent large glaucoma treatment trials have used different criteria to define it.

Confirmatory testing

In the great majority of clinical situations there will be time for a confirmatory visual-field test. It is important to be certain of progression before acting upon it. This is important prior to considering commencement or alteration of treatment but is of paramount importance before embarking upon surgery. Clinical practice suggests that patients need at least two or three repeat visual-field tests before a diagnosis of progression can be made with any confidence.

The Ocular Hypertension Treatment Study (OHTS) has recently highlighted and characterized this point. The study authors evaluated the frequency with which patients who had been identified as reaching a pre-specified visual-field end-point (based upon the glaucoma hemifield test) subsequently had a normal visual field.[5] At the commencement of the study two consecutive, reliable, abnormal visual fields were required to deem that progression to glaucoma had occurred (one of the end-points of this study). When they used the original plan of two consecutive visual fields to confirm progression to glaucoma, two thirds of these patients amazingly had a subsequent normal visual field. This means that in 66% of cases, despite two visual fields which reached a hard-and-fast threshold for definition of glaucoma, the finding only occurred because of those patients' LTF. Whereas if three consecutive visual fields were needed to confirm a field defect only 12% of patients had a subsequent visual field which returned to normal. This third visual-field test significantly reduced the number of future visual-field tests that improved back to baseline. The OHTS protocol was subsequently changed, requiring three consecutive, abnormal and reliable visual-field tests for a patient to reach the glaucoma end-point.

The Advanced Glaucoma Intervention Study (AGIS)[6] also helped with the understanding of visual field fluctuation. Patients had an eligibility visual-field test at the time they were enrolled

(a) CENTRAL 24-2 THRESHOLD TEST

FIXATION MONITOR: BLINDSPOT   STIMULUS: III. WHITE   PUPIL DIAMETER: DATE: 20-10-2005

FIXATION TARGET: CENTRAL   BACKGROUND: 31.5 ASB   VISUAL ACUITY: TIME: 16:04

FIXATION LOSSES: 0/10   STRATEGY: SITA-FAST   RX: +4.50 DS   DC   X   AGE: 79

FALSE POS ERRORS: 0 %

FALSE NEG ERRORS: 4 %

TEST DURATION: 02:56

FOVEA: 35 DB

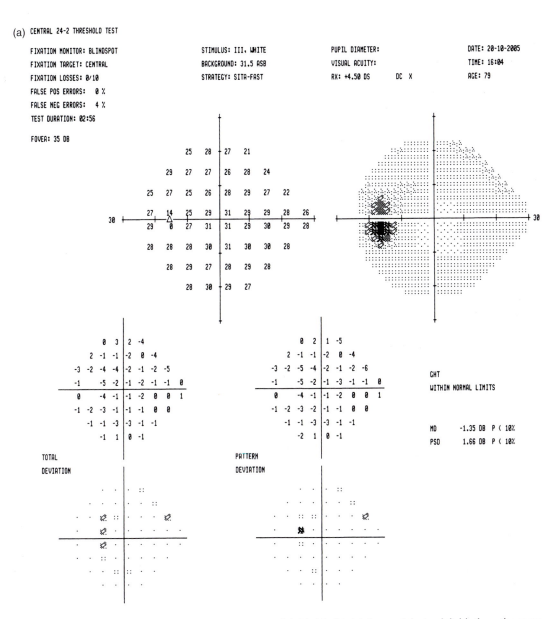

Figure 13.1 Visual-field fluctuation. Need for repeat visual field. (a), (b), (c) Sequential visual fields from the same patient. Each visual field has reasonable reliability. The second visual field is markedly worse than the first, with a significant visual-field defect. A further visual-field assessment reveals that the field defect has disappeared. This highlights the need for confirmatory visual fields before making a decision on progression.

(b)

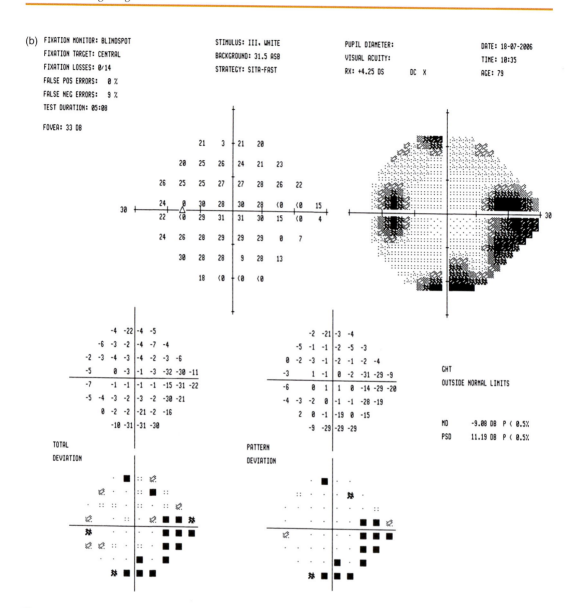

FIXATION MONITOR: BLINDSPOT
FIXATION TARGET: CENTRAL
FIXATION LOSSES: 0/14
FALSE POS ERRORS: 0 %
FALSE NEG ERRORS: 9 %
TEST DURATION: 05:08

FOVEA: 33 DB

STIMULUS: III. WHITE
BACKGROUND: 31.5 ASB
STRATEGY: SITA-FAST

PUPIL DIAMETER:
VISUAL ACUITY:
RX: +4.25 DS   DC   X

DATE: 18-07-2006
TIME: 10:35
AGE: 79

GHT
OUTSIDE NORMAL LIMITS

MD   -9.08 DB P < 0.5%
PSD   11.19 DB P < 0.5%

TOTAL
DEVIATION

PATTERN
DEVIATION

Figure 13.1 (Continued)

(c) CENTRAL 24-2 THRESHOLD TEST

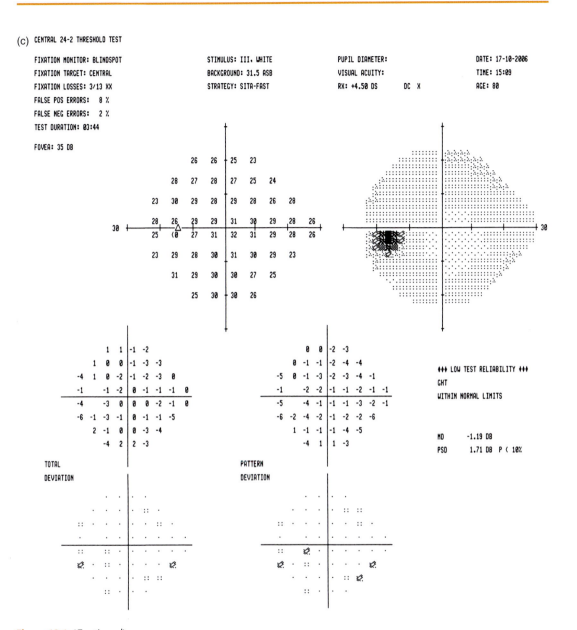

FIXATION MONITOR: BLINDSPOT
FIXATION TARGET: CENTRAL
FIXATION LOSSES: 3/13 XX
FALSE POS ERRORS: 0 %
FALSE NEG ERRORS: 2 %
TEST DURATION: 03:44

FOVEA: 35 DB

STIMULUS: III, WHITE
BACKGROUND: 31.5 ASB
STRATEGY: SITA-FAST

PUPIL DIAMETER:
VISUAL ACUITY:
RX: +4.50 DS   DC X

DATE: 17-10-2006
TIME: 15:09
AGE: 80

TOTAL DEVIATION

PATTERN DEVIATION

✦✦✦ LOW TEST RELIABILITY ✦✦✦
GHT
WITHIN NORMAL LIMITS

MD   -1.19 DB
PSD   1.71 DB P (10%

Figure 13.1 (Continued)

and a pre-intervention visual-field test before the intervention to lower IOP. More than 12 000 visual fields from 565 patients were evaluated. When comparing the eligibility and the pre-intervention field tests, 5% of the eyes tested significantly worse on the latter test and 11% tested better. When they analyzed this further they found that significant visual-field improvement was less likely for eyes with mild visual-field defect scores (4%) compared with eyes with moderate (11%, $P = 0.013$) or severe (17%, $P = 0.005$) visual-field defect scores. So, rather annoyingly, the patients with the worst visual field tended to have the greatest level of fluctuation.

One study suggested that it takes approximately 5 years of follow-up with annual perimetry before you can detect significant changes in the visual field.[7]

Glaucoma change probability analysis

The Humphrey visual-field analyzer has an inbuilt piece of software which aims to help the clinician decide if progression is occurring. The glaucoma change probability analysis (GCPA) is the statistical software that evaluates visual-field change over time based upon the total deviation plot. The statistical database contains information about a group of non-progressive glaucoma eyes. It checks each point on the visual field and works out whether that has changed to the previous fields. If change is detected it scrutinizes the depths and patterns of these changes and compares them with its stable database. The stable group would have had some physiological variation in their repeat fields (their LTF) and this degree of variation is taken to be the 'normal' threshold of LTF. A change in the patient's visual field that exceeds this threshold LTF is felt to represent true deterioration and not simply fluctuation. Points with significant deterioration are displayed as black triangles while areas of improvements are shown as white triangles.

One problem with the GCPA is that it is does not focus on the pattern deviation plot and thus media opacities or miotic pupils may affect its results. One other flaw with the GCPA database is that it was based upon patients who were experienced and consistently reliable in automated perimetry and who underwent four visual-field tests in only a 1-month period. In clinical practice patients are often far from experienced and reliable in perimetry and the visual fields are much further apart meaning that comparison to this database is not truly 'like with like'. The GCPA database concentrates on patients with moderate defects and thus using it to analyze patients with severe or mild defects may lead to inaccuracy due to inherent differences in physiological LTF between these groups.

Finally patients are individuals and have individual levels of LTF. Attributing a one-size-fits-all LTF to all patients is problematic. The GCPA does what the clinician should be methodically doing anyway. However, the clinician has the benefit of having the serial visual fields from their patient before them thus facilitating comparison to that patient's individualized LTF.

Progression by expansion or deepening of a scotoma

It makes intuitive sense that areas of glaucoma damage represent susceptible areas and that as damage worsens these areas would be affected more and more. Thus as glaucoma progresses it seems logical that is does so by deepening and expansion of an existing scotoma. Clinical practice would suggest that this is indeed the case and one study[8] conducted work to directly assess this concept. They used specific defined criteria to identify progression and then carefully examined sequential visual fields for evidence of this. Interestingly none of their patients progressed by developing a new scotoma.

Thus it is important to focus attention on existing areas of field defect either formally by testing that area only (for example carry out 10-2 visual fields only on a paracentral scotoma) or by the clinician consciously looking at the precise values within and adjacent to an existing defect.

Quantitative assessment

Theoretically we could extend the utility of the GCPA and develop a piece of software or artificial intelligence to do the work for us and detect progression. Previous studies on neural network's ability to detect glaucoma progression have been encouraging but we have not been replaced just yet.[9,10]

Researchers have used pointwise linear regression (PLR) to evaluate visual-field progression with some success.[11] Regression slopes were considered clinically and statistically significant if they measured more than −1 dB/year. These strategies tended to concentrate on consistent changes in GHT clusters within a visual field series. In order to get good PLR values, six to eight visual fields are required.

Despite all the clever technologies currently the best way to assess for visual-field progression is to sit down with the sequential visual fields and examine them yourself.

The patient is older every time they repeat their visual-field test and thus the likelihood of deteriorated central acuity due to macula pathology or media opacity is greater. Development of visually significant cataracts can make the detection of progression difficult as it can mask focal defects as well as mimic the overall depression caused by advanced disease. Techniques that analyze pattern deviation plot results should control for the presence of media opacity, however, this can be falsely controlled for true overall depression. It is the clinician's responsibility to double check the visual fields and the clinical picture in order to make sure that true progression is picked up and false progression due to other factors is detected.

Clinical examination for progression

In clinical practice no clever technology replaces the clinician in evaluating the visual fields to pick up progression. When assessing a series of visual fields you are asking two questions. Has an OHT patient progressed to glaucoma or has a patient with established glaucoma progressed?

Organization is invaluable for the assessment of visual fields. Print out all the available visual fields and group all the right and left eyes. This will save a considerable amount of time and will prevent confusion. Next take one eye and line the visual fields up. Make sure that they are all of the same patient and place them in chronological order. Scan their reliability indices. Group them into reliable, borderline reliable and absolutely unreliable ('hopeless'!). The hopeless visual fields should be put to one side as they convey little information and can make interpretation harder than if the patient had not those tests done at all.

To review a series of fields rapidly for progression obtain a print-out in an overview format which displays the grayscale, threshold values, total deviation plots and pattern deviation plots on a single line. The GHT analysis, reliability indices and global indices are also listed for each field. Up to three fields can be displayed on a single page, which allows an easy scan of the elements of the display and ready assessment of trends. This display does not analyze the information for progression but simply lays out the data in a convenient format for scrutiny by you.

Adjacent to the grayscale are the more important threshold values. It is logistically impossible to compare the threshold values for every single point on every single plot. It is thus more appropriate to concentrate on areas highlighted on the grayscale to determine whether newly developed areas of reduced sensitivity are truly present (and representative of glaucoma) or whether pre-existing defects are widening and/or deepening.

The clinician has to decide how much the sensitivity thresholds have to reduce before the results can be considered true progression rather than simply a manifestation of LTF.

Examine sequential pattern deviation plots for progression. Before making decisions look at the total deviation plots and compare them to the pattern deviation plots. Is there a marked difference? If so does the patient have a clinical reason for reduced sensitivity across the board? Confirm they have some degree of cataract or miosis to account for any difference seen. When the whole field worsens by the same degree it is hard to differentiate true overall diffuse glaucoma progression from a worsening due to increased media opacity (remember that cataracts get worse with time!).

As previously highlighted when a point dips into the $p < 0.05$ level the probability plot shows a black square. Any more deterioration at that point results in no further change in the appearance of the probability plot. A point can lose 20% of its sensitivity and show up as a black square on the probability plot for a decade and then progress to complete loss of sensitivity (absolute scotoma) without any hint of worsening appearing on the probability plot. Again it is vital to look at the absolute figures on the pattern deviation plot to see how a scotoma is changing. A reliable and repeatable drop from −10 dB to −32 dB clearly breaches the patient's LTF and is a manifestation of progression. The statistical package which produces the statistical plot is helpful in highlighting the development of glaucoma or detecting progression in early glaucoma but tends to be less helpful once established field defects are present as seen in moderate to advanced glaucoma.

Before you decide whether the patient has progressed it is important to consider what you are comparing to. You need a baseline. Naturally in an ocular hypertensive who is a reliable visual field producer the baseline is a normal visual field. In established glaucoma the baseline is often generated by their first couple of visual fields. Changes in the patient will affect this baseline.

If progression is detected and the patient undergoes a change in management to attain a lower target IOP, be it surgical or medical intervention, then the new baseline becomes the progressed field and not the original field. It will probably take several visual fields to establish this new baseline. It should also be noted that the visual fields in the months after the attainment of the new target IOP may actually continue to progress as they may be manifesting damage which has occurred before the IOP was lowered. Once the new baseline series of visual field are obtained (usually two or three) all further visual fields are compared to that new baseline.

If a patient is noted to have diffuse progression and it is felt that this may be due to a cataract then the patient may be a good candidate for consideration of cataract surgery if appropriate. If the patient does have cataract surgery then the first few visual fields after the surgery will form the new baseline for future comparison.

If treatment is initiated in a new glaucoma patient then the baseline visual field may not be the first one they do for several reasons. They will be at the start of their learning curve and so even if the reliability indices are reasonable they may have some scope for improvement. The clinician cannot hope to understand a patient's LTF with only one visual field. At least two or three are required to understand the patient's baseline 'range' of visual fields. Finally, as mentioned previously, the first few visual fields may potentially reflect damage that occurred before they presented with their untreated IOP.

Once an area of the field has been identified as possibly having progressed, the clinician has to decide whether this change is significant enough to warrant a change in management, usually in the hope of achieving lower IOP.

Progression is unlikely to occur in only one point. A 10 dB loss of sensitivity in one point is usually accompanied by a 5 dB loss in one or more adjacent points. This makes logical sense and emphasizes the need to examine the numbers within and adjacent to a scotoma to detect evidence of progression. It is sensible to examine visual fields as a series of zones of normality or abnormality and observe changes within those zones.

If there was no detriment then it would make sense to repeat visual fields five or six times in order to confirm progression before changing management. Unfortunately if patients are progressing then they will continue to lose visual field while the clinician deliberates as to whether the field has, and is, continuing to progress. The need to intervene should be balanced with the risks of that intervention. In general it is sensible to seek two confirmatory 'worse' visual fields before initiating a change in medical treatment. Naturally it is vital to confirm that the apparent worsening is consistent with the rest of the clinical picture, for example changes in the disc in the appropriate place and a raised IOP.

The more inconsistencies in the clinical picture the more confirmatory tests are required. For example in a patient with an apparently minimally cupped disc with only marginal NRR thinning and an IOP of 10 mmHg (and a normal CCT) any apparent progression has to be questioned as it 'doesn't make sense' in the context of the favorable clinical picture. Naturally such patients may have another cause for their visual-field loss and an index of suspicion has to be maintained in such cases that the clinician is missing a pathology, be it retinal, optic nerve or intracranial.

If invasive surgical intervention is contemplated, with all the inherent risks therein, it makes sense to obtain three confirmatory visual fields if there is any doubt about the progression demonstrated in the first two. Naturally the rate of progression will have a bearing on how much time you have to play with. If progression is apparently rapid (consistent and fitting with the clinical picture) then the need for confirmatory visual fields may be negated both because you are reasonably confident that there is indeed progression and because of a relative urgency to reduce the IOP and prevent further loss.

In the presence of suspected progression repeat visual fields should not be delayed inappropriately. Follow-up testing and clinical assessment should be carried out in accordance with the index of suspicion of progression. In a patient with equivocal evidence of maybe slight progression and an IOP reaching the previously established target IOP, a confirmatory test can wait 3–4 months. In a moderately advanced glaucoma patient with an IOP above a previously set target and a significantly deepening scotoma close to fixation, a repeat confirmatory visual field may be appropriate within a few weeks.

Identifying progression in end-stage glaucoma

Picking up progression in advanced glaucoma is often harder than detecting it in early or moderate glaucoma. This is a significant problem as patients with advanced disease have very little reserve and even a slight degree of loss may jeopardize central acuity or result in other forms of immediately noticeable visual morbidity.

A patient with end-stage glaucoma needs monitoring with 10-2 visual fields as 24-2 and 30-2 visual-field test points are too far apart to allow adequate monitoring of the points close to fixation. If the patient does still have some residual visual field remaining out of this 10° area it can be checked by a 30-2 visual field using a size V stimulus instead of the standard size III. If the patient is so advanced that they do not produce enough responses for meaningful interpretation using the normal 10-2, a size V stimulus can be used instead, in the hope of gaining a field which can subsequently be used as a baseline to detect progression.

In patients with end-stage disease the aim is to preserve central acuity. Typically, the superior nasal field progresses inward to split fixation, followed by loss in the inferior field that encroaches from the nasal field as well.[12]

References

1. Heiji A, Lindgren A, Lindgren G. Test-retest variability in glaucomatous visual fields. Am J Ophthalmol 1989; 108: 130–135.
2. Werner EB, Petrig B, Krupin T, Bishop K. Variability of automated visual fields in clinically stable glaucoma patients. Invest Ophthalmol Vis Sci 1989; 30: 1083–1089.
3. Boeglin RJ, Zulauf M, Hoffman D, *et al*. Long-term fluctuation of the visual field in clinically stable glaucoma patients. Invest Ophthalmol Vis Sci 1991; 32: 1192–1198.
4. Henson DB, Spry PG, Spencer IC, Sparrow JM. Variability in glaucomatous visual fields: implications for shared care schemes. Ophthalmic Physiol Opt 1998; 18: 120–125.
5. Keltner JL, Johnson CA, Levine RA, Fan J, Cello KE, Kass MA, Gordon MO. Normal visual-field test results following glaucomatous visual field end points in the Ocular Hypertension Treatment Study. Arch Ophthalmol 2005; 123: 1201–1206.
6. Kim J, Dally LG, Ederer F, Gaasterland DE, VanVeldhuisen PC, Blackwell B, Sullivan EK, Prum B, Shafranov G, Beck A, Spaeth GL; AGIS Investigators. The Advanced Glaucoma Intervention Study (AGIS): 14. Distinguishing progression of glaucoma from visual field fluctuations. Ophthalmology 2004; 111: 2109–2016.
7. Smith SD, Katz J, Quigley HA. Analysis of progressive change in automated visual fields in glaucoma. Invest Ophthalmol Vis Sci 1996; 37: 1419–1428.
8. Boden C, Blumenthal EZ, Pascual J, McEwan G, Weinreb RN, Medeiros F, Sample PA. Patterns of glaucomatous visual field progression identified by three progression criteria. Am J Ophthalmol 2004; 138: 1029–1036.
9. Brigatti L, Nouri-Mahdavi K, Weitzman M, Caprioli J. Automatic detection of glaucomatous visual field progression with neural networks. Arch Ophthalmol 1997; 115: 725–728.
10. Sample PA, Boden C, Zhang Z, *et al*. Unsupervised machine learning with independent component analysis to identify areas of progression in glaucomatous visual fields. Invest Ophthalmol Vis Sci 2005; 46(10): 3684–3692.
11. Nouri-Mahdavi K, Caprioli J, Coleman AL, Hoffman D, Gaasterland D. Pointwise linear regression for evaluation of visual field outcomes and comparison with the advanced glaucoma intervention study methods. Arch Ophthalmol 2005; 123: 193–199.
12. Weber J, Schultz T, Ulrich H. The visual field in advanced glaucoma. Int Ophthalmol 1989; 13: 47–50.

Chapter 14

Identifying progressive morphological change

Why should I read this chapter?

We now know how to detect visual-field progression, however the visual field loss is permanent and irreversible. It would be better if we could determine progression without having to sacrifice any visual field at all. It is accepted that there is often a lag between morphological change and visual-field change. If we can pick up structural change early we may be able to prevent any visual-field loss at all by intervening early. New imaging devices are promising tools for this function but unfortunately they have significant weaknesses which the clinician needs to fully understand.

Identifying progression

Worsening of optic disc cupping and the development of localized neuroretinal rim loss are key features of glaucoma progression. Detecting these changes early and altering treatment expeditiously should help to prevent progression. Changes in the optic disc and RNFL are a key feature of glaucoma and play a vital role in the diagnosis. Patients progress by both structure and function, but these are not necessarily identified at the same time.

Landmark work by Quigley carried out many years ago suggested that up to 50% of the ganglion cell axons can be lost before kinetic perimetry detects a visual-field defect.[1] Automated static perimetry does slightly better, but up to 20–40% of the axons can still be lost before a field defect manifests.[2] This data suggests that morphological changes precede visual-field loss and that should we be able to detect these structural changes early enough we may be able to prevent the subsequent visual-field loss.

It must be remembered however that this spare capacity applies for each bit of the nerve and not the nerve as a whole. In the event of a localized notch in the disc it may take only a 30% loss of nerve fiber layer in that clock-hour to begin to manifest an arcuate visual-field defect. This 30% loss in one small area may represent a minute loss of ganglion cells when considering the whole eye, but in this small area the damage has worsened enough to result in functional loss. With more loss in that area the visual-field defect will rapidly worsen as all redundancy is already gone. Even small changes in nerve fiber numbers will manifest as progressive field loss.

Quantification of disc damage has always been a key concern. Historically this has relied on physical examination and documentation of morphological characteristics in the clinical notes.

The CDR has been a steadfast tool in our armamentarium when discussing glaucomatous change of the optic nerve head. We know that as glaucoma worsens the cupping of the optic disc also worsens. This is one of the hallmarks of glaucoma. The exact pattern and pathogenesis of NRR loss in glaucoma is not categorically established, however it is clear that NRR area declines over time in untreated glaucoma patients. One group of researchers[3] assessed the rate and pattern of NRR area decrease in normals, OHT and glaucoma. Rim area loss was linear in 49% of the patients, episodic in 22% and curvilinear in 29%. The yearly loss of rim area was 0.23% of the initial area in normal subjects, 0.47% and 2.75% in the patients with stable and deteriorating ocular hypertension, respectively, and 3.47% in the patients with deteriorating glaucoma. It is interesting to note that normal patients also lost NRR area over time, thus indicating that normal physiological changes are occurring and we have to contend with these also when looking for progression.

One of the major mainstays of glaucoma progression detection is serial assessment of the ONH and RNFL. Clinical examination is still the best way to detect progressive structural changes however objective quantitative assessment is difficult. Several modern devices have been developed to aid the clinician in ONH and RNFL evaluation.

Quantitative structural assessment of the optic nerve head and RNFL with modern imaging devices provides an objective, reproducible and reliable measure of optic disc structure and ganglion cell axons. Quantitative assessment with imaging devices augments (but does not replace) the subjective evaluation of patients at the slit lamp. While potentially of help in screening for gluacoma, arguably the greatest benefit of newer imaging devices is in the objective and quantitative monitoring of glaucoma and the identification and quantification of progression.

To repeat a continually recurring theme it is important to understand that any devices cannot replace the clinician and examining the optic nerve head and RNFL with your own eyes is still the gold standard in care. If technology is used the clinician using it should understand its limitations and its potential strengths. Clinicians make decisions on progression by interpreting clinical data, only one part of which are the results of the various imaging devices.

Measuring the rate of progression

As well as giving evidence of progression, devices may also provide information regarding the rate of damage. This can have significant implications as regards the type and extent of intervention required to arrest the patient's glaucoma.

Progression may be monitored by either event analyses or by trend analyses. Event analysis is defined as the breaching of a predetermined threshold of change. Trend analysis looks at the change in a measurement over time. A measured rate of progression may help in the assessment of a patient's lifetime risk of developing functionally significant visual loss.

Morphological predictive factors for development or progression of glaucomatous visual-field defects in white people are a small neuroretinal rim area (i.e. advanced glaucoma) and a large beta-zone of parapapillary atrophy.[4]

Optic disc photographs

Optic disc photography is the oldest form of optic disc imaging and it still has its uses in modern practice. ONH photographs can be monoscopic, sequential stereoscopic or simultaneous stereoscopic. Simultaneous stereoscopic photography is the best as, when viewed with stereo viewers, a three-dimensional impression of the disc may be obtained and a true assessment of the optic cup and NRR can be obtained.[5] This allows the clinician to compare the appearance they see before them when they examine the patient to the previous picture. Other features such as increasing peripapillary atrophy and disc hemorrhages[6–8] can also be seen clearly and documented in photographs.

Optic disc photography has tended to be superseded by other forms of technology mainly due to the poor availability of appropriate viewing systems. Print-outs of the photographs are time consuming and use lots of consumables. In addition viewing of photographs on a print-out or on a computer screen without stereo facilities does not give an optimal impression of the true disc morphology. There is technology available which allows viewing of stereoscopic photographs in three dimensions on the computer screen but it is not in widespread use.[9,10]

Studies looking at assessing glaucoma progression from serial optic disc photographs usually use expert observers with specialized tailored equipment which of course does not represent the true situation in day-to-day clinical practice.

If logistically possible it makes sense to obtain optic disc photographs when the glaucoma patient first presents. Ideally these photographs should be stereo, however even mono-digital images using modern cameras can give a wealth of information. Making diagnoses or deciding progression purely based upon two-dimensional images is inadvisable, however, being able to look back at previous disc appearance is invaluable. Optic disc photographs can also help in engaging the patient in their disease by showing them exactly what we are looking at and why we are concerned for them.

The need for standardized, reproducible and digitalized optic disc imaging has spurred numerous advances in technology. Photographic optic disc imaging techniques have largely been superseded by digital scanning devices such as scanning laser tomography (SLT), scanning laser polarimetry (SLP) and optical coherence tomography (OCT). The technology is moving forward so quickly that very little long term follow-up data exists for the currently available devices making precise guidance as to long-term utility in the follow-up situation difficult.

Scanning laser tomography

SLT delivers surface three-dimensional topographic data from a stack of confocal images of the ONH. An observer draws around the ONH margin to allow calculation of parameters such as cup and rim. The most commonly used commercially available device is the Heidelberg Retina Tomograph (HRT) (Heidelberg Engineering, Germany).

Studies have shown that rim area is the most repeatable optic nerve head parameter measured using the HRT. Research has been undertaken to examine the test–retest variability of the stereometric parameter measures made with the HRT, and which values provide the most repeatable and reliable measurements.[11] NRR area and mean cup depth measurements have been found to be least variable pieces of data. Their consistency and repeatability means that any changes should (theoretically) represent real alteration in optic nerve head morphology, thus indicating that sequential rim area measurements by HRT may be ideal for monitoring glaucomatous progression.

In addition the ability to discriminate between normal and glaucomatous eyes[12] and the inherent measurement repeatability of HRT[13,14] makes it a good candidate for progression detection.

As previously detailed, progression can be identified by 'event' analysis or with a 'trend' analysis. The SLT provides data at the pixel level and also within the calculated parameters.

Change analysis may be applied to the individual pixels[1-3] or to the produced parameters.[15-18] In event analysis, progression is identified when a measurement difference exceeds a preset threshold. This threshold may be determined from measurement variability in images acquired from the same eyes either in the same session[16,19] or on different occasions,[17] or from variability in the sequential results of an unchanging (normal or non-progressing) reference group.[18] Event analysis is less than ideal in the clinical setting of glaucoma management. Of more use is the detection of a pattern of deterioration – i.e. a trend analysis. This also has the bonus of furnishing us with an idea of rate of progression which can have implications on our management decisions. It can also give an idea of how our interventions change the rate of deterioration even if we do not arrest it completely.

One of the simplest ways to use the HRT for detection of progression is to scrutinize the numerous stereometric parameters presented. The progression print-outs can provide you with a graph of the various parameters over time. It is important to set the print-out to provide you with specific information. The default setting is to provide you with progression of the global indices. This takes everything and jumbles it all up into one number. It is clearly useless. It is important to set it to NRR which is really the best parameter to scrutinize when looking for change. If the patient is perimetric it is important to correlate any changes in the NRR with the visual field. OHT patients may be noted to have progressive thinning of the NRR before they display field loss.[19]

The other feature of the HRT is the topographic change analysis (TCA). This is a statistical method which compares the topographic height values in groups of pixels over time. The TCA works out statistical likelihood of real change in the height values in these groups. The standard deviation (SD) of the individual scans will have a significant effect on how well the TCA functions. If the SD is large then there is clearly a lot of noise and it will struggle to detect progression unless the change in topography height is marked.

TCA is automatically performed when there is one set of baseline images and at least two sets of follow-up images. The main analysis from TCA is presented in the form of the change probability maps (Fig. 14.1). The reflectivity maps are overlaid with red and green symbols that highlight areas in red where the loss of height is significant. Areas in green show areas of elevation.

The TCA is sensitive to poor image alignment and also struggles when the image qualities are poor. It also remains unclear as to when this demonstrated loss of topographic height becomes clinically significant. It is unknown how many clusters of red squares need to be seen before a patient with OHT needs treatment. In clinical practice it makes sense that if there is suspected progression of a superior arcuate scotoma and the TCA brings up a massive cluster of red squares in the inferior portion of the nerve head that we take this at face value and settle on a diagnosis of progression.

As with all the imaging devices they need to be used with caution until they are truly validated and specific guidelines may be offered. All the clinical parameters must be taken into account before decisions are made. Look for corroborating evidence.

Scanning laser polarimetry

This technology uses a scanning laser ophthalmoscope to analyze the change in polarization in light reflected from the fundus and equates this (after correction for anterior segment polarization) to RNFL thickness.

We know that RNFL is lost before a visual-field defect manifests. As clinicians we can visualize the optic disc ourselves and should be able to spot a worsening notch or increasing CDR.

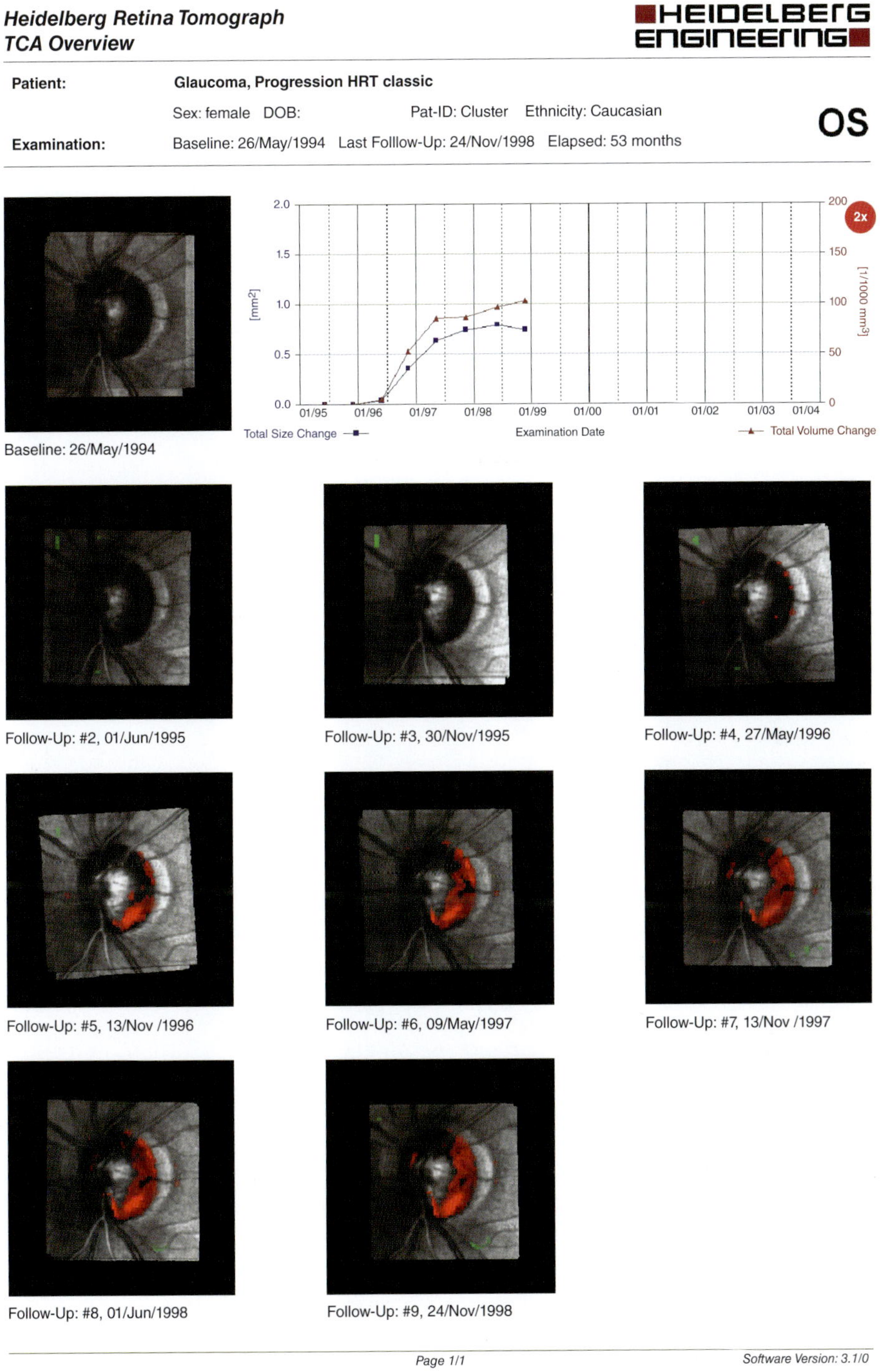

Figure 14.1 HRT Change Probability Map. This shows a single display with all reflectivity and topography images in the series. Areas of significant neuroretinal rim loss are highlighted in red.

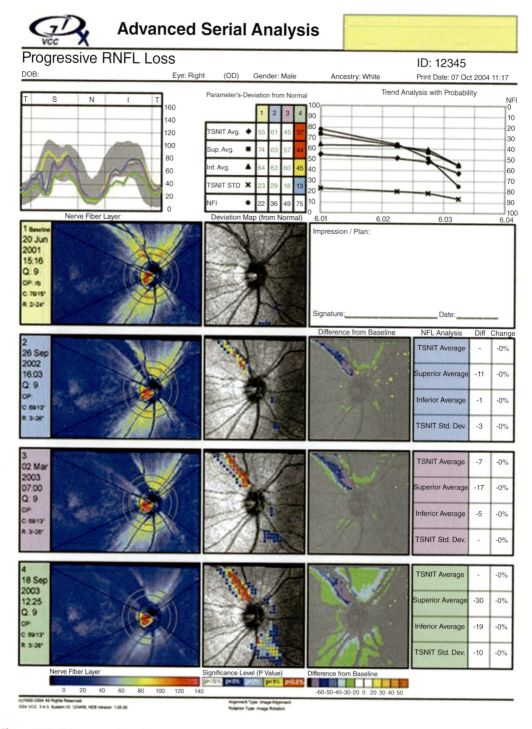

We do not stand a chance, however, of picking up gradual loss of RNFL. Monitoring of local RNFL changes over time with the GDx VCC sounds like an ideal way of detecting progression early.

The NFI index has been shown to be good at discriminating between glaucoma and normality. Observing a change in the NFI over time may give a clue as to worsening in RNFL parameters. For example, an OHT patient with a normal NFI initially which gradually creeps towards abnormality over time may give us a clue as to potential conversion to glaucoma. The progression analysis component of the GDx VCC software quantifies local change and displays it in a color-coded probability map (Fig. 14.2).

The use of the GDx for serial assessment of glaucoma is as yet unproven. It appears to be a promising tool, but formal validation is required before definitive guidance can be offered.

Optical coherence tomography

OCT is based on low coherence interferometry and acquires cross-sectional images through the retina with very high depth resolution (up to 10 μm). The technique identifies interfaces between the different layers of the retina, including the anterior and posterior borders of the RNFL thus providing thickness data. RNFL thickness measurements by OCT discriminate well between normal and glaucomatous eyes and are highly reproducible, thus theoretically making it a good tool for detection of progression.

There is very little data available on the use of RNFL OCT to monitor for progression of glaucoma. The follow-up print-out (Fig. 14.3) displays the change in RNFL thickness compared

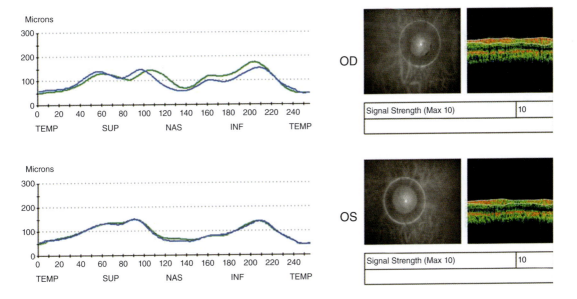

Figure 14.3 OCT RNFL progression.

to the previous scans for each point. Where the line dips below the horizontal it indicates loss of RNFL thickness. In clinical practice this is highly dependent upon image quality. Poor image quality makes these follow-up assessments virtually useless.

Longitudinal studies are required before we can fully assess its utility.

Summary

It can clearly be seen that there is no ideal tool for monitoring progression. It sounds like a great idea but inter-test variability tends to be the Achilles heel of all these devices. The changes in glaucoma are subtle with a loss of microns of tissue, be it NRR or RNFL, potentially representing significant glaucoma progression. In an ideal world we have to pick up this structural change early, before the visual field worsens. Otherwise we may as well wait for the visual-field deterioration and simply use the imaging devices as an adjunct to confirm progression rather than using it to help us prevent the visual-field progression. Time will allow for validation of these devices. Of the three devices HRT and GDx seem the most promising for this arena.

References

1. Quigley H, Addicks E, Green W. Optic nerve damage in human glaucoma. III. Quantitative correlation of nerve fiber loss and visual-field defect in glaucoma, ischemic optic neuropathy, disk edema, and toxic neuropathy. Am J Ophthalmol 1983; 673–679.
2. Quigley H, Dunkelgerger B, Green W. Retinal ganglion cell atrophy correlated with automated perimetry in human eyes with glaucoma. Am J Ophthalmol 1989; 107(5): 453–464.
3. Airaksinen PJ, Tuulonen A. Alanko HI. Rate and pattern of neuroretinal rim area decrease in ocular hypertension and glaucoma. Arch Ophlhalmol 1992; 110: 206–210.
4. Jonas JB, Martus P, Horn FK, Junemann A, Korth M, Budde WM. Predictive factors of the optic nerve head for development or progression of glaucomatous visual field loss. Invest Ophthalmol Vis Sci 2004; 45: 2613–2618.
5. Boes DA, Spaeth GL, Mills RP, Smith M, Nicholl JE, Clifton BC. Relative optic cup depth assessments using three stereo photograph viewing methods. J Glaucoma 1996; 5: 9–14.
6. Rasker MT, Van den Enden A, Bakker D, Hoyng PF. Deterioration of visual fields in patients with glaucoma with and without optic disc hemorrhages. Arch Ophthalmol 1997; 115: 1257–1262.
7. Drance S, Anderson DR, Schulzer M. Risk factors for progression of visual field abnormalities in normal-tension glaucoma. Am J Ophthalmol 2001; 131: 699–708.
8. Uchida H, Ugurlu S, Caprioli J. Increasing peripapillary atrophy is associated with progressive glaucoma. Ophthalmology 1998; 105: 1541–1545.
9. Barry CJ, Eikelboom R, Kanagasingam Y, *et al*. Comparison of optic disc image assessment methods when examining serial photographs for glaucomatous progression. Br J Ophthalmol 2000; 84: 28–30.
10. Morgan JE, Sheen NJ, North RV, *et al*. Discrimination of glaucomatous optic neuropathy by digital stereoscopic analysis. Ophthalmology 2005; 112: 855–862.
11. Tan JC, Garway-Heath OF, Hitchings RA. Variability across the optic nerve head in scanning laser tomography. Br J Ophthalmol 2003; 87: 557–559.
12. Wollstein G, Garway-Heath DF, Hitehings RA. Identification of early glaucoma cases with the scanning laser ophthalmoscope. Ophthalmology 1998; 105: 1557–1563.

13. Sihota R, Gulati V, Agarwal HC, *et al.* Variables affecting test-retest variability of Heidelberg Retina Tomograph II stereometric parameters. J Glaucoma 2002; 11: 321–328.

14. Strouthidis NG, White ET, Owen VM, *et al.* Factors affecting the test-retest variability of Heidelberg retina tomograph and Heidelberg retina tomograph II measurements. BrJ Ophthalmol 2005; 89: 1427–1432.

19. Chauhan BC, Blanchard JW, Hamilton DC, LeBlanc RP. Technique for detecting serial topographic changes in the optic disc and peripapillary retina using scanning laser tomography. Invest Ophthalmol Vis Sci 2000; 41: 775–782.

15. Artes PH, Chauhan BC. Longitudinal changes in the visual field and optic disc in glaucoma. Prog Retina Eye Res 2005; 24: 333–354.

16. Tan JC, Poinoosawmy D, Hitchings RA. Tomographic identification of neuroretinal rim loss in high-pressure, normal-pressure, and suspected glaucoma. Invest Ophthalmol Vis Sci 2004; 45: 2279–2285.

17. Burgoyne CF, Mercante DE, Thompson HW. Change detection in regional and volumetric disc parameters using longitudinal confocal scanning laser tomography. Ophthalmology 2002; 109: 455–466.

18. Kamal DS, Garway-Heath DF, Hitchings RA, Fitzke PW. Use of sequential Heidelberg retina tomograph images to identify changes at the optic disc in ocular hypertensive patients at risk of developing glaucoma. Br J Ophthalmol 2000; 84: 993–998.

19. Kamal DS, Viswanathan AC, Garway-Heath DF, Hitchings RA, Poinoosawmy D, Bunce C. Detection of optic disc change with the Heidelberg retina tomograph before confirmed visual field change in ocular hypertensives converting to early glaucoma. Br J Ophthalmol 1999; 83: 290–294.

Section 3

Management of glaucoma

So far we have achieved a level of competence in discriminating glaucoma from normality and we also have a handle on how to detect progression of glaucoma. We need to proceed now into how we manage our patients with glaucoma. This is a general guide and should act as a starting point in your glaucoma management. Gradually as your skills evolve and your experience builds you will develop your own treatment algorithms. It is important to maintain your training throughout your glaucoma career and maintain links with the hospital and the glaucoma specialist you are allied with.

Patients are individuals and so these generalizations cannot be applied to all patients. Each case should be managed according to the specific clinical characteristics.

Chapter 15

Target IOP

Why should I read this chapter?

Target IOP is in my opinion a vital tool in the glaucoma clinician's armamentarium. It is not utilized by everyone and some people feel that it is a pointless exercise. If we are managing patients by bringing their IOPs down it is important that we know what we are aiming for. By keeping a handle on this we can see whether we achieved our aim (or target!) and also whether we drift away from it with the passage of time. The pressure we need could be assessed at every visit but this would entail looking back through the visual fields every time and checking the pattern of IOP since the patient presented. It seems to make sense to do this thoroughly and methodically on one occasion and get an idea of what IOP you would be happy at running the patient at. This is a dynamic tool and can be changed – it is only a starting point. Use it and see if you find it valuable.

Introduction

'The target IOP is the IOP at a certain point in an eye's diurnal IOP curve at which it is felt that the progression of the patient's glaucomatous optic neuropathy will not result in significant patient specific visual morbidity in that patient's lifetime. Achievement of target IOP should take into account the risk versus benefit profile for any intervention designed to achieve it.' *Catchy definition, eh*!

When assessing a glaucoma or ocular hypertensive patient it is important that the clinician has an idea of the target IOP. Literally what are we aiming for? At what IOP do we sit back and say that we have achieved our goal? At what level of IOP do we strive to do more to bring the pressure down?

It is important that there is some flexibility with regards target IOP. A one-off reading 1 mmHg above target IOP in a patient on maximal medical therapy should not immediately trigger listing for surgery.

Reaching documented target IOP should allow the clinician to confidently say that the patient's IOP is satisfactory and no further intervention is required *at that time point*. Naturally this depends upon a static visual field and an unchanging optic disc.

Failure to attain target IOP should cause the clinician to address the patient's glaucoma control in depth. Attainment of a target IOP but evidence of progression means that the target IOP was not set low enough. In addition it should prompt the clinician to consider the diurnal curve of IOP and in particular to reflect on the effect of IOP fluctuation on glaucoma progression.

A target IOP may be moved up as well as down. In the absence of any documented progression it is reasonable to move a patient's target IOP up to a higher level if the attainment of their original target IOP may put the patient at risk.

It is my belief that target IOP should be documented in each and every glaucoma and ocular hypertensive patient; however, this view is contentious. Target IOP is a powerful tool however and, as with every tool, it is not infallible. If used, it is important that the clinician fully comprehends the ethos of it and factors involved in defining it.

The above definition is broken down into its components below.

'The target IOP is the IOP at a certain point in an eye's diurnal IOP curve'

As previously emphasized it is important that the IOP is documented at a specific time point. We know that treating a patient will lower their whole diurnal IOP curve. It is also well established that glaucoma filtering surgery will result in significant flattening of diurnal IOP fluctuation.[1] The target IOP may not actually represent the IOP at which no further damage occurs. It may simply represent lowering of the whole diurnal curve so that the peak diurnal IOP point now lies below the damage line.

Clinical example

A 56-year-old patient had documented visual-field progression with 9–10 am IOP readings of 18 mmHg on one medication. A target IOP is subsequently set at 15 mmHg and a further drop added to achieve this. A follow-up IOP measured at 4 pm is 18 mmHg, clearly breaching the target IOP. This may still be acceptable: the IOP at which the damage occurred was actually 22 mmHg at 4 pm, when the IOP was repeatedly measured at between 9 and 10 am to be 18 mmHg. By treatment we have brought the whole diurnal curve down and the patient is no longer spiking up to 22 mmHg and suffering damage at this IOP (Fig. 15.1).

'at which it is felt'

Naturally the target IOP set is based upon the clinician's best judgment. There are no hard-and-fast guidelines or formulae which dictate what target IOP should be set. This will be dependent upon the pre-treatment IOP and also the degree of glaucomatous damage at baseline. It may be set too high, requiring revision to a lower level if further deterioration

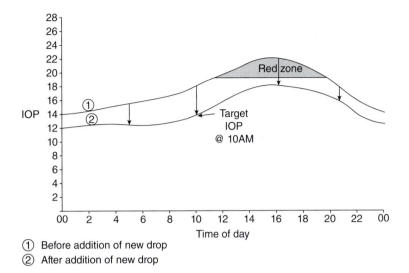

① Before addition of new drop
② After addition of new drop

Figure 15.1 Lowering whole diurnal curve by treatment. Graph showing the patient's diurnal IOP curve. (1) Pre-treatment. (2) After addition of extra drop. We can see that the whole IOP curve has been lowered and the patient no longer enters the theoretical red zone of damage.

occurs or it may be revised to a higher level if the risk–benefit profile of actively attaining it is unjustified.

'that the progression of the patient's glaucomatous optic neuropathy will not result in significant patient specific visual morbidity'

It is not always necessary that the attainment of target IOP should herald no further glaucomatous deterioration. While this is ideal, it is impossible in some circumstances to safely attain an IOP which would arrest glaucomatous progression entirely. Different patients have different visual needs. Naturally patients still driving will find it paramount that their visual field is maintained enough so that they may still drive. Patients who rely on driving for their livelihood will be even more motivated to maintain their level of visual field above the critical level.

'in that patient's lifetime'

Different patients will live for differing lengths of time. Interventions to bring IOP down may be inappropriate if the likelihood is that the anticipated loss of visual field will result in no visual morbidity in that patent's lifetime. In elderly patients with persistent slow progression at target IOP and limited life expectancy it may not be necessary to lower their target IOP at all. Conversely a younger patient will have many years of life ahead and thus early arresting of glaucomatous progression will be paramount.

'Achievement of target IOP should take into account the risk versus benefit profile for any intervention designed to achieve it'

This is an important facet of the target IOP ethos. The benefits in the form of slowing glaucomatous progression and subsequent prevention of visual morbidity must be balanced against the risks of the treatment aimed at achieving it. The addition of a drop to achieve target IOP is a relatively minor intervention with a well documented safety profile. In the setting of maximal medical therapy, if the target IOP is not achieved and laser therapy is inappropriate then surgical intervention is the logical next step. The potential complications of surgical intervention are not negligible and thus the risks of this intervention have to be balanced carefully against the likely benefit in prevention of glaucoma progression.

If the IOP attained is within a few mmHg of target it may be reasonable to observe the rate of glaucoma progression and then make judgments upon it at that stage. Observation of rate of change should give some indication as to the likelihood of morbidity should further IOP lowering not be achieved. It is vital that any decisions regarding risks and benefits of intervention be discussed at great length with the patient themselves. After all it is their visual ability we are predicting and should surgery be undertaken it is their vision we are gambling against the risk of potential complication.

Setting a target intraocular pressure

The goal of all glaucoma treatment is to maintain vision so that patients can maintain enough visual function to allow them to perform their desired visual tasks throughout the rest of their lives. In addition we must aim to limit the side effects of therapy and (particularly in this day and age of health economic constraints) minimize or optimize costs of glaucoma treatment.

Most patients with mild to moderate glaucoma damage are generally asymptomatic and can function visually without compromise. The goal of treatment in these patients is not necessarily to halt glaucoma progression totally but to slow the rate of progression to such a degree that we are able to keep the patient visually functional in their daily occupational and personal lives.

Patient age at diagnosis is also very important in determining the aggressiveness of therapy required. Younger patients diagnosed with glaucoma have more years to become visually impaired from their disease and warrant more aggressive treatment than an elderly patient presenting with the same degree of damage. A slow rate of progression may have no effect on an 80-year-old with a life expectancy of 10 years however in a 30-year-old this same slow rate of worsening may lead to blindness in their early 60s.

Each glaucoma patient behaves differently. One patient may never progress again after lowering their IOP by 30% while another with exactly the same starting IOP and the same IOP reduction may progress rapidly. The patient's target pressure must be continually reassessed at every visit and potentially adjusted based on the presence or absence of glaucomatous progression.

Once a diagnosis of glaucoma has been made and the patient has had baseline IOP measurements taken (including a baseline diurnal curve if logistically possible), the clinician must decide what target IOP to set as a starting point. In general, the greater the amount of damage present at presentation (based upon the visual field and the optic disc appearance) the greater the percentage of IOP lowering required.

As a general guide, patients with mild visual field loss require 20–30% IOP reduction; with moderate loss, 30–40% IOP reduction; and with severe loss, 40–50% IOP reduction. Of course patients with a mild visual-field defect but an almost fully cupped optic disc (assuming it is of normal size) may warrant greater pressure reduction than that outlined above, emphasizing the need for individualized targets based upon all the clinical features of the patient.

A patient's presenting IOP should also have a bearing upon the target IOP set. If a patient presents with a pressure of 50 mmHg then a 30% reduction down to 35 mmHg may not be enough, especially if the patient's disc is markedly compromised. Such a patient would probably benefit from at least a 50% reduction of IOP down to 25 mmHg or lower (see text below). Conversely it may be excessive to aim for a 50% pressure reduction in a patient with mild glaucoma and a presenting IOP of 26 mmHg.

Other determinants of target pressures include the race of the patient and any family history of blindness from glaucoma. Black patients are more likely to show progression of their disease than age-matched white patients, and patients with a definitive family history of blindness from glaucoma or a sibling with glaucoma also warrant more aggressive therapy and a lower initial target IOP (see Chapter 2).

A patient who has only one seeing eye, is unable to perform reliable visual-field testing, or has other optic nerve or retinal diseases likely to affect the ability to follow the patient for progression are all indicators for more aggressive treatment.

Clinically setting target IOP

New patient

The diagnosis of glaucoma has been established by clinical examination and visual-field assessment. It has been elected to treat the patient and now, as the treating clinician, you need to set an initial target IOP.

One simple method of determining an initial target IOP is to take the presenting IOP (or the highest IOP reading taken during follow-up) and note that numerical value. Next take the mean deviation of the visual field and add that numerical value to that of the highest IOP. Add an extra 5 for specific risk factors such as black ethnicity, young patient age and uniocularity and then use this new value to determine the percentage IOP reduction required to achieve the target IOP.

For example, taking the patients described earlier:

- Patient 1. Presenting IOP 50 mmHg and severe visual-field defect with a mean deviation of −21 dB. A target IOP may be set in this patient of 50 + 21 = 71% IOP reduction, i.e. 35.5 mmHg pressure drop with a target IOP of 14.5 mmHg, target IOP < 15 mmHg. If the patient is uniocular a pressure reduction of around 75% may be sought.
- Patient 2. Presenting IOP 26 mmHg and mild visual-field defect with a mean deviation of −5 dB. A target IOP may be set in this patient of 26 + 5 = 31% IOP reduction, i.e. 8 mmHg pressure drop with a target IOP of less than 18 mmHg. If the patient were black, a 5% supplemental IOP reduction may be prudent.

Again it has to be emphasized that the above rules are generalizations and should not be used blindly.

A patient under follow-up who has demonstrated progression

Here it is important to identify at what IOP the glaucoma progressed. Thorough examination of the patient records is vital to determine a time scale for the deterioration. In the majority of cases this progression will be reasonably slow. We must ask ourselves at what IOP or, more likely, IOP range did this progressive damage occur? We must also bear in mind that we will be judging the IOP based upon solitary readings with no account taken of any diurnal fluctuation.

If we see damage which occurred over a period of 2 years during which time the IOP varied between 18 mmHg and 22 mmHg (always measured in the morning) we can take the midpoint of those readings as a baseline IOP at which the glaucoma was uncontrolled. Next we must assess the rapidity of this worsening. Theoretically the further we are above the target IOP the faster the progression will occur. If the IOP is only a few mmHg above target IOP then the patient should only progress slowly. If the patient's IOP is well in excess of target IOP then the progression will be rapid. Thus we can use the rate of the progression as a yard stick for how far from target IOP the patient is. As a general rule a further 15–20% reduction in IOP is desirable. If the progression is rapid then a 30% or even 40% further reduction may be required.

How do we reach a target IOP?

Currently we have medical therapy, laser therapy and surgical intervention in our armamentarium. Each has its own place in glaucoma management with very different efficacy and risk profiles. The patient must be actively involved in the decision-making process before embarking upon a management strategy.

Reference

1. Konstas AG, Topouzis F, Leliopoulou O, Pappas T, Georgiadis N, Jenkins JN, Stewart WC. 24-hour intraocular pressure control with maximum medical therapy compared with surgery in patients with advanced open-angle glaucoma. Ophthalmology 2006; 113: 765.

Chapter 16

Glaucoma medications

Why should I read this chapter?

Most of your glaucoma patients will be on glaucoma medications. It is vital to know how they work and the problems that can occur with their use. Before commencing treatment you have to understand what conditions are contraindicated to avoid doing any harm to the patient. Different drugs have different roles to play. Gradually you will develop your own hierarchy of treatment as your experience grows.

Anatomy of aqueous dynamics

Aqueous is continually produced by active secretion from the ciliary body and flows into the posterior chamber (PC) at a rate of a few microliters per minute. To balance this there is continual aqueous outflow from the AC resulting in complete turnover of aqueous volume every 1–2 hours.

Beta-adrenergic agonist activity is thought to play a role in the active aqueous secretory process, hence the therapeutic effects of adrenergic blockade. Beta-blockade of the ciliary body, mainly through beta-2-receptors, reduces the amount of aqueous production, while activation of the alpha-receptors, also found on the ciliary body, results in decreased aqueous production.

Aqueous moves from the PC into the AC through the pupil. It has to flow from the ciliary body across the surface of the lens and pass through the pupil to eventually reach the drainage angle. Aqueous provides the vital metabolic and nutritional needs to the avascular lens and cornea. Approximately 80% of aqueous exits the eye through the trabecular meshwork (TM) into Schlemm's canal (SC) and then into the episcleral venous plexus. The juxtacanalicular trabecular meshwork is the key membrane in controlling the rate of aqueous outflow and it is thought that changes in this membrane are responsible for reducing outflow capacity and causing glaucoma.

TM outflow is a pressure-dependent mechanism. At raised IOPs the TM distends and aqueous outflow is facilitated, lowering IOP. This mechanism is pharmacologically utilized by cholinergic stimulation of the ciliary muscle causing the ciliary body to contract and stretch open the TM.

Up to 20% of aqueous outflow from the eye is via the pressure-independent uveoscleral pathway. This pathway is not distinct in anatomical localization. It encompasses absorption of aqueous by the ciliary body and iris and passage of aqueous through the longitudinal muscle fibers of the ciliary body directly into the suprachoroidal space. The advent of synthetic prostaglandin analogs which facilitate increased uveoscleral outflow has highlighted the importance of this aqueous outflow mechanism.

Rate of aqueous production is not constant. Aqueous production has a range in healthy patients from 1.8–4.3 μl/minute; the rate is generally highest in morning hours, slightly lower during the afternoon hours, and approximately one-half of the morning rate during sleep.[1] The rate declines by 3.2% per decade after the age of 10 years, and there is no gender difference.[2] Several researchers have documented IOP spikes on awakening lasting approximately 30 minutes.[2,3] Wide diurnal variations occur more frequently among glaucoma patients than non-glaucoma patients.[4–6]

An understanding of the mechanisms of aqueous production and outflow opens up numerous therapeutic avenues for increasing this outflow and lowering IOP. Numerous medications have been developed which lower IOP to differing degrees. It should be remembered that generalization is impossible and different patients will respond with a different efficacy and side-effect profile.

Anti-glaucoma agents

Beta-adrenergic blocking agents

Such medications may be selective, targeting one specific beta-adrenergic receptor, or they may be non-selective having a broad effect on all adrenergic function within the eye.

Timolol maleate

This is a non-selective beta-blocking agent that has no preference for beta-1- or beta-2-receptors. Timolol reduces aqueous production via an effect on the beta-receptors of the ciliary body. The majority of patients will achieve a 20% reduction in IOP. There is a small group of patients who do not respond to this drug. Its effectiveness can diminish during the first 2 weeks by approximately 30–40% (short-term escape) and further slight loss of efficacy can occur within about the first 3 months (long-term drift).

As the drug has significant systemic absorption the other eye is also affected when only one eye is treated. Information gleaned from the Glaucoma Laser Trial[7] suggested a 0.5 mmHg contralateral effect. However, other work[8] has suggested this may be more in the region of 3 mmHg.

Timolol is historically one of the most commonly prescribed beta-blocking agents. It is cheap, effective and, in the majority of patients, safe. Timolol is available in two concentrations: 0.25% and 0.5%. The 0.25% concentration has similar efficacy to the stronger concentration with fewer systemic side effects and so should be the drop of choice when using timolol.

Timolol LA

Timolol LA is the long-acting variant of timolol and allows for once-daily rather than twice-daily dosing. It is also available in 0.25% and 0.5% concentrations. Its long-lasting effect is brought about by the special vehicle which changes from a liquid to a gel-like state when it is instilled and should thus give 24-hour IOP-lowering coverage.

Levobunolol (Betagan)

Levobunolol is a non-selective beta-blocker that has similar IOP-lowering effect and systemic side-effect profile to timolol. It is available as 0.25% and 0.5% solutions. The 0.5% solution instilled once daily should give the same efficacy as the 0.25% solution applied twice a day.

Side effects and contraindications of non-selective beta-blockers

Beta-blockers have an excellent efficacy profile, but their major problems are related to their systemic side effects. Beta-receptors are present throughout the body with high concentrations of the beta-1-receptor found on the heart, and beta-2-receptors on the bronchioles of the lungs. Side effects most frequently occur in patients who have some form of chronic obstructive pulmonary disease (COPD), such as chronic bronchitis, emphysema or asthma.

Beta-blockers prevent bronchial smooth muscle relaxation by blocking receptor sites thus resulting in narrowed airways and shortness of breath. Patients with congestive cardiac failure, bradycardia (defined as a resting heart rate lower than 60 beats per minute) or heart block may suffer exacerbation of their condition with the use of topical beta-blockers. Patients already on some form of systemic beta-blockade or calcium channel blocker therapy should be monitored for potential additive toxicity. If the clinical need is great then consultation should be sought with the patient's cardiologist, respiratory physician or general practitioner before commencing these medications in at-risk patients. Patients with risk factors for adverse events should ideally be managed with other forms of medication. Should beta-blockers be used, consider obtaining formal written consent explaining clearly the risks of commencement or continuation of such drops. Ocular side effects are relatively rare and include stinging, dry eye and hyperemia.

Betaxolol (Betoptic, Betoptic S)

With concerns about systemic toxicity and the side effects of indiscriminate beta-blockade, attempts have been made to create selective beta-blockers to target specific receptors and spare others.

Betaxolol is a beta-1 selective blocker. It has roughly similar efficacy to timolol and because of its relative cardiac specificity it is theoretically less likely to induce any respiratory side effects. Despite this theoretical safety benefit it is still inadvisable to use any topical beta-blockers in patients with significant respiratory disease. Of course cardiac conditions are contraindications as in the case of the non-selective beta-blockers.[9]

Clinical use of beta-blockers

Beta-blockers have been the first line therapy for glaucoma for many years. Their position of primacy has been superseded to some degree by the prostaglandin analogs which are now arguably the best first-line treatment for glaucoma.

When using these drugs it is prudent to take and more importantly document any history (or lack thereof) of cardiac or respiratory contraindications to beta-blocker use. It is also wise to take a resting pulse rate to ensure the patient does not have a pre-existing bradycardia.

These drops may lose efficacy with time thus giving the patient the risks of complication without the benefits of IOP reduction. In patients on long-term beta-blocker therapy there is the potential that they have completely lost efficacy. In such situations it may be worthwhile stopping the drops temporarily to assess their true effect (if any) on IOP. A uniocular drug cessation trial may be appropriate but it is worthwhile remembering that uniocular beta-blockers also have a contralateral effect.

Adrenergic agonists

Apraclonidine (Iopidine)

Apraclonidine is an alpha-2 adrenergic blocker which lowers IOP by decreasing aqueous production at the ciliary body. It has the ability to lower IOP within 1 hour of instillation, with an effect which lasts at least 12 hours. A concentration of 1% was able to produce up to a 37% reduction in IOP, and the 0.5% concentration produced an average decrease in IOP of 27%.[10–14] It is available as a 1% concentration in a unit dose ampoule (0.5 ml) and as a 0.5% solution in a 5 ml bottle.

Side effects and contraindications of apraclonidine

Apraclonidine has little effect on the cardiovascular and pulmonary systems but can cause problems with dry mouth (occuring in approximately 20–50% of patients) and sedation (in up to 10% of patients[10,15]). Despite the above, the systemic side effects tend to be tolerable. The real problem with the medication are the ocular side effects, the major one being the incidence of allergic reaction and tachyphylaxis. Allergic conjunctivitis occurs in 9% of patients within 3 months of use, and in almost half of patients on longer-term therapy.[12,16,17] The drug also suffers from a relatively short period of efficacy with tachyphylaxis often occurring after only a few months of use.[18,19]

Indications for apraclonidine

Apraclonidine main use is in the prevention of IOP spikes following anterior segment laser procedures. It is also a useful drug when rapid acute pressure reduction is required, for example in a patient with PAC.[20] Its use in glaucoma management is limited by the adverse ocular tolerability profile and the relatively rapid loss of efficacy when used for longer-term treatment. It may have a role in patients already on maximal medical therapy where surgery is deemed to be high risk, however, such patients should be closely monitored to detect allergy or tachyphylaxis.

Brimonidine (Alphagan)

Brimonidine is an excellent alpha-2-receptor agonist. Brimonidine is less prone to oxidation than apraclonidine and is thus less prone to inducing allergy.[21] Brimonidine lowers IOP by decreasing aqueous production and by increasing uveoscleral outflow.[22]

Brimonidine 0.2% administered twice daily was found to be comparable to timolol 0.5% and superior to betaxolol.[23–25]

Animal studies are available that suggest that brimonidine exhibits neuroprotective properties. The first such study by Lair and colleagues demonstrated the drug's ability to protect rat neurons from injury.[26] The second, by Mitchell and associates, used rabbit retinal ganglion cells. The drug inhibited glutamate-mediated injury.[27] The jury is still out regarding the true 'neuroprotective' potential of this drug and certainly no *in vivo* clinical evidence exists to support such a claim.

Side effects and contraindications of brimonidine

The most common side effects of brimonidine are ocular irritation, allergy and blurring of vision. Allergy occurs in as many as 10% of patients on long-term therapy.[28] Fatigue, dry mouth, sedation and reduction of systemic blood pressure are the most significant systemic problems associated with brimonidine. Brimonidine cannot be used in infants or children because of reported episodes of syncope, or in patients taking MAO inhibitors.

Clinical use of alpha-adrenergic agonists

These are useful drugs in the anti-glaucoma armamentarium. Due to the ocular side-effect profile and the incidence of tachyphylaxis they tend to be used as a third-line regimen. Primary use of these medications is not advised. The use of apraclonidine to prevent IOP spikes is a firm niche and its efficacy and tolerability is clear in this setting. Use of brimonidine for chronic therapy is usually well tolerated and, as long as regular review is ensured, then it can always be stopped/ switched if intolerance develops with no long-term detriment.

Cholinergic agents

These compounds reduce IOP by stimulation of the ciliary muscle, which pulls on the TM and increases the outflow of aqueous as previously described. Cholinergics are very effective in lowering IOP in the majority of patients. Naturally should the TM be damaged cholinergics are less effective. They are additive to beta-blockers, carbonic anhydrase inhibitors (CAIs) and alpha-agonists, however they may inhibit uveoscleral outflow thus negating some prostaglandin-induced IOP reduction. They also induce miosis which may be used as a marker for compliance but more often results in adverse patient symptoms.

In PAC, miotics help to pull the peripheral iris away from angle structures assuming that peripheral anterior synechiae have not yet formed.

Pilocarpine

Pilocarpine is available in various concentrations (0.5%, 1%, 2%, 3%, 4%) and is usually administered four times a day due to its short duration of action. Low concentrations (such as 1 or 2%) of pilocarpine are often used for therapeutic miosis, for example in situations where the patient has potentially occludable angles and is awaiting laser peripheral iridotomy.

When used therapeutically in OAG it seems prudent to slowly increase the dosage in stepwise increments to minimize the incidence of adverse patient symptoms. In general a maximum concentration of 2% is used in patients with light-colored irides, while in brown or dark irides, a maximum concentration of 4% should be used.

Cholinergic side effects and contraindications

Cholinergic therapy is contraindicated in uveitic, neovascular and other secondary angle-closure glaucomas.

Due to the induced miosis patients may experience peripheral and night vision problems. Patients with a centrally located lens opacity or posterior subcapsular cataract may experience a significant reduction in vision due to pupil miosis. Patients may also experience brow pain and accommodative spasm after the use of pilocarpine. The pain usually occurs within a few minutes and lasts on average 15–20 minutes. The accommodative spasm and induced myopia make such drugs unsuitable for pre-presbyopic patients.

Ciliary muscle contraction pulls on the TM but it also applies traction to the pars plana potentially exacerbating any pre-existing retinal traction and potentially causing retinal breaks or even causing a retinal detachment.

Chronic pilocarpine use can result in a small pupil which is less and less amenable to pharmacological mydriasis. This can be particularly troublesome in patients who have other disorders such as peripheral retinal degenerations or diabetic retinopathy and require regular retinal examination. A particularly miosed pupil can even make formal disc assessment virtually impossible.

Systemic side effects of cholinergic agents include gastrointestinal upset, salivation, abdominal cramping and potential heart block.[29] Toxicity is usually related to overall dosage and frequency of administration. Pouring pilocarpine on to an eye in PAC and a markedly raised IOP may precipitate significant systemic toxicity without any effect on pupil size.

Clinical use of cholinergic agents

With the advent of newer therapies the use of miotic agents has lessened significantly. The side-effect profile is generally unacceptable in the great majority of patients and thus it should be reserved for patients already on maximal medical therapy if surgery is contraindicated.

Topical carbonic anhydrase inhibitors (CAIs)

Carbonic anhydrase inhibitors decrease aqueous production by inhibiting the enzyme, carbonic anhydrase, a key part of the pathway of aqueous production at the ciliary body.

Topical carbonic anhydrase inhibitors

Dorzolamide (Trusopt)

Topical CAIs do not work as well as oral CAIs (see below) mainly due to their poor corneal penetration. Dorzolamide 2% is given as a three times daily dose if used without concurrent topical beta-blockers or twice daily if topical beta-blockers are also used. Dorzolamide achieves an approximately 20% reduction in IOP.[30,31]

Brinzolamide (Azopt)

Brinzolamide 1% (Alcon, Fort Worth, TX) is another topical CAI and is used in a twice daily dosage. The use of a suspension form allows the drug to be buffered at physiologic pH hopefully making it a much more comfortable drug to use than its cousin Trusopt. Brinzolamide is equivalent in IOP-lowering effect to dorzolamide.[32]

Side effects and contraindications of topical carbonic anhydrase inhibitors

Side effects include mild hyperemia, ocular stinging and a bitter taste in the mouth. The two latter complications are more pertinent to the dorzolamide preparation rather than the brinzolamide. The stinging is due to the fact that dorzolamide must be buffered at the acidic pH of 5.6. The drugs should not be used in patients with sensitivity to sulfonamide drugs.

Clinical use of topical carbonic anhydrase inhibitors

These drugs are usually well tolerated and efficacious. They tend to be used as a second- or third-line medication when target IOP has not been reached with mono- or dual therapy. There is a theoretical problem in patients with pre-existing corneal decompensation or Fuchs' endothelial dystrophy as carbonic anhydrase is an important enzyme in the endothelial corneal pump which maintains the cornea's state of relative dehydration. Clinicians should be cautious about using topical CAIs in patients with such pre-existing corneal pathologies. Pachymetry may be used to detect any adverse effects on corneal thickness.

Oral carbonic anhydrase inhibitors

Acetazolamide (Diamox)

CAIs represent a very effective method of lowering IOP, with reductions of as much as 35%.[33] Acetazolamide is available in 125 mg or 250 mg tablets, or 250 mg slow-release capsules. The maximum dosage is 1 gram in 24 hours. The slow-release preparation should negate some of the adverse side effects of the medication.

Systemic side effects and contraindications of oral carbonic anhydrase inhibitors

Carbonic anhydrase is an enzyme in numerous metabolic pathways throughout the body and thus it is unsurprising that systemic side effects are commonly encountered with use of oral CAIs. The most notable side effects include paresthesia (tingling of the hands and feet), malaise, gastrointestinal disturbance and polyuria. Renal function can be severely affected over a long course of treatment due to metabolic effects and also due to the presence of induced kidney stones and degenerative glomerular changes. Other side effects of CAIs include anorexia, metabolic acidosis, and alterations in mental status (depression, psychosis or mental confusion).

Hypokalaemia (potassium depletion) is a significant problem with CAIs, especially in hypertensive patients using non-potassium-sparing diuretics. Low serum potassium may result in fatal cardiac complications and should be considered and tested for in such patients on long-term therapy. If necessary, liaison with the patient's cardiologist or general practitioner is prudent.

Aplastic anemia is a potentially fatal blood dyscrasia, where the bone marrow stops producing red and white blood cells, and platelets. It is a rare complication of oral CAIs, but it appears to be an idiosyncratic reaction, with no way to predict which patients are at risk.

Lastly, acetazolamide is contraindicated in pregnant women during the first trimester and probably throughout the whole of pregnancy and breast feeding. Although it has never been shown to produce teratogenicity in humans, it has produced limb deformities in rats.[34]

Clinical use of systemic carbonic anhydrase inhibitors

Despite the numerous downsides to oral CAI treatment there is no doubt that they are extremely effective in lowering IOP. The number of effective topical medications available mean that the use of oral CAIs for chronic management of glaucoma is not common. They are invaluable in the management of acute pressure rises and for prophylaxis against pressure spikes after certain forms of surgery.

Some patients tolerate systemic CAIs extremely well and they may chose to stay on them rather than proceed to higher-risk interventional procedures to lower IOP.

Prostaglandin agents

Prostaglandins are arguably the best topical drop for IOP reduction. They are well tolerated, efficacious and benefit from once-daily dosing. These compounds significantly reduce IOP by increasing uveoscleral outflow.

There are three available preparations: latanoprost (Xalatan, Pfizer), travoprost (Travatan, Alcon) and bimatoprost (Lumigan, Allergan). They share a common biochemical nature in that they are all prostaglandin PGF2alpha agonists and increase uveoscleral outflow facilitating about a 30%+ drop in IOP from baseline.

Side effects and contraindications of prostaglandin analogs

Prostaglandin analogs have little effect on systemic cardiovascular and respiratory function. Ocular side effects include stinging, tearing and conjunctival hyperemia. Hyperemia tends to be mild but can be significant enough to discontinue the medication. These drugs may induce irreversible darkening of the iris by increasing melanin within the iris melanocytes. They also cause lash growth which is often seen as an added bonus to younger female patients. Patients on unilateral prostaglandin therapy may experience significant asymmetry of ocular appearance and they should be warned of this.

There is much controversy regarding the role and use of prostaglandin analogs in cases of cystoid macular edema and anterior uveitis. Aphakic and pseudophakic patients with posterior capsule breaks appear to be at greatest risk. Because of the potential exacerbating effect of prostaglandins on uveitis, they should, in general, be avoided in the presence of ocular inflammation.

Clinical use of prostaglandin analogs

These are excellent drugs and are extremely effective at lowering IOP. They are also generally well tolerated both systemically and ocularly. Once-daily dosing, proven efficacy and tolerability make these drugs a powerful tool for use against glaucoma.

They should generally be used as first-line therapy in the majority of routine patients. There is a proportion of patients who do not respond to these medications and thus the use of monocular drug trials seems prudent when initiating treatment to detect the true IOP-lowering efficacy.

Hyperosmotic agents

Osmotic agents reduce IOP by reducing vitreous volume. They do this by increasing plasma osmolality thereby 'sucking' water out of the vitreous cavity. Unfortunately these agents also pull fluid into the intravascular space from every part of the body resulting in potential systemic problems. They also stimulate a brisk and rapid diuresis which may be detrimental in the elderly, infirm or those with comorbidity.

These agents are not for chronic use and their effect is very short term. They are reserved to treat a single event of highly elevated IOP found in either open- or narrow-angle glaucoma.

Glycerin

This oral hyperosmotic agent is given in a 50% solution and produces an average vitreous body shrinkage of 3–4%[35], potentially facilitating an IOP reduction of more than 30 mmHg.

This osmotic agent should be ingested rapidly to maximally change osmolality and produce an effect. Patients often experience severe nausea when they take this drug and serving it over ice may help overcome this and prevent the patient vomiting the drug up.

Glycerin is broken down to glucose, and thus it should be used with extreme caution in diabetic patients.

Mannitol

Due to the problems in keeping the glycerin down most patients achieve a better clinical response if intravenous mannitol is used. It tends to be the drug of choice because it does not penetrate into the vitreous cavity thus enhancing its osmotic mode of action. The recommended dosage of mannitol is 7.5–10.0 ml/kg of a 20% solution. The drug has to be given quite rapidly for full effect. Within about half an hour renal excretion is enhanced and the patient experiences a marked diuresis.

Side effects and contraindications of hyperosmotic agents

Extreme caution should be used with these agents, especially in the elderly population. The rapid increase in intravascular volume followed by an equally rapid depletion results in significant stress on the patient's cardiovascular system as it increases output to compensate for a decreased blood and tissue volume. This additional stress could produce cardiac failure.

Clinical use of hyperosmotic agents

These potent agents are not appropriate for long-term use. They should only be used when a rapid pressure reduction is required when the IOP is dangerously high. Such agents are frequently used in the management of attacks of PAC. Patients should be closely monitored and extreme caution should be used in the elderly or those with cardiovascular comorbidity.

Combination drops

There are numerous combination drugs available. The use of two drops in one has theoretical benefits of improving patient compliance and decreasing the preservative load upon the eye.

Cosopt: timolol and dorzolamide combination

Cosopt is a combination of 0.5% timolol and 2% dorzolamide. Studies show a similar IOP lowering with Cosopt prescribed twice daily with separate dosing of 0.5% timolol twice a day and 2% dorzolamide twice a day.

Combigan: timolol and brimonidine combination

Combigan is a combination of 0.5% timolol and 0.2% brimonidine.

Beta-blocker and prostaglandin combination

There are three combination drops which contain a prostaglandin analog and 0.5% timolol. They are Xalacom (Xalatan/Timolol), DuoTrav (Travatan/Timolol) and GanForte (Lumigan/Timolol). As part of their approval process all of these drugs have had to demonstrate non-inferiority to the separate drops.

Clinical use of combination drops

Combination drops should not be used as first-line therapies. Combination drops should be used when the patient has not achieved enough of a pressure reduction on monotherapy alone.

Naturally the cost profile for combination drops should be balanced against the potential improved patient complicance and convenience.

(See Chapter 17 for details of clinical utility of combination drops.)

References

1. Brubaker RF. Flow of aqueous humor in humans (The Freidwald Lecture). Invest Ophthalmol Vis Sci 1991; 32: 3145.
2. David R, Zangwill L, Briscoe D, *et al*. Diurnal intraocular pressure variations: an analysis of 690 diurnal curves. Br J Ophthalmol 1992; 76: 280.
3. Zeimer RC, Wilensky JT, Gieser DE. Presence and rapid decline of early morning intraocular pressure peaks in glaucoma patients. Ophthalmology 1990; 97: 548.
4. Brown B, Burton P, Mann S, Parisi A. Fluctuations in intra-ocular pressure with sleep: II. Time course of IOP decrease after waking from sleep. Ophthalmic Physiol Optics 1988; 8: 249.
5. Wilensky JT. Diurnal variations in intraocular pressure. Trans Am Ophthalmol Soc 1991; 89: 757.
6. Henkind P, Walsh JB. Diurnal variations in intraocular pressure. Chronic open angle glaucoma: preliminary report. Aust J Ophthalmol 1981; 9: 219.
7. The GLT Laser Trial Research Group. The Glaucoma Laser Trial (GLT): results of argon laser tra-beculoplasty. Ophthalmology 1990; 97: 1403.
8. Dunham CN, Spaide RF, Dunham G. The contralateral reduction of intraocular pressure by timolol. Br J Ophthalmol 1994; 78: 38–40.
9. Kirwan JF, Nightingale JA, Bunce C, Wormald R. Do selective topical beta antagonists for glaucoma have respiratory side effects? Br J Ophthalmol 2004; 88: 196–198.
10. Abrams, DA, Robin AL, Crandall AS, *et al*. A limited comparison of apraclonidine's dose response in subjects with normal or increased intraocular pressure. Am J Ophthalmol 1989; 108: 230.
11. Abrams DA, Robin AL, Pollack IP, *et al*. The safety and efficacy of topical 1% apraclonidine in normal volunteers. Arch Ophthalmol 1987; 105: 1205–1207.
12. Nagasubramanian S, Hitchings RA, Demailly P, *et al*. Comparison of apraclonidine and timolol in chronic open-angle glaucoma. A three month study. Ophthalmology 1993; 100: 1318.
13. Lee DA, Topper JE, Brubaker RE. Effect of clonidine on aqueous humor flow in normal human eyes. Exp Eye Res 1984; 38: 239–246.
14. Butler P, Mannschreck M, Lin S, *et al*. Clinical experience with the long-term use of 1 % apracloni-dine. Arch Ophthalmol 1995; 13: 293.
15. Morrison JC, Robin AL. Adjunctive glaucoma therapy: a comparison of apraclonidine to dipivefrin when added to timolol maleate. Ophthalmology 1989; 96: 3–7.

16. Stewart WC, Ritch R, Shin DH, *et al.* The efficacy of apraclonadine as an adjunct to timolol therapy. Arch Ophthalmol 1995; 13: 287–292.
17. Butler PJ, Jones B. Incidence of characteristics of allergic reaction to apraclonidine 0.5%. Invest Ophthalmol Vis Sci 1996; 37: S201.
18. Cardakli F, Smythe B, Eisele J, *et al.* Effect of chronic apraclonidine treatment on intraocular pressure in advanced glaucoma. J Glaucoma 1992; 1: 271–278.
19. Lish A, Camras C, Podos S. Effect of apraclonidine on intraocular pressure in glaucoma patients receiving maximally tolerated medication. J Glaucoma 1992; 1: 19–22.
20. Krawitz PL, Podos SM. Use of apraclonidine in the treatment of acute angle-closure glaucoma. Arch Ophthalmol 1990; 108: 1208.
21. Toris CB, Tafoya ME, Cambras CB, *et al.* Effects of aproclonidine on aqueous humor dynamics in human eyes. Ophthalmology 1995; 102: 456–461.
22. Toris CB, Cambras CB, Yablonski ME. Effects of brimonidine on aqueous humor dynamics in human eyes. Arch Ophthalmol 1995; 113: 1514–1517.
23. Schuman JS. Clinical experience with brimonidine 0.2% and timolol 0.5% in glaucoma and ocular hypertension. Surv Ophthalmol 1996; 41: S27–S37.
24. Schuman JS, Horwitz B, Choplin NT, *et al.* A one year study of brimonidine twice daily in glaucoma and ocular hypertension. A controlled, randomized, multicenter clinical trial. Arch Ophthalmol 1997; 15: 847–852.
25. Javitt J, for the Brimonidine Outcome Study Group. The clinical success rate and quality of life assessment of brimonidine tartrate 0.2% compared with timolol 0.5% administered twice-daily, in patients with previously untreated open-angle glaucoma or ocular hypertension. Invest Ophthalmol Vis Sci 1997; 38: S729.
26. Lai R, Hasson D, Chun T, Wheeler L. Neuro-protective effect of ocular hypotensive agent brimonidine. XIth Congress of the European Society of Ophthalmology Proceedings 1997, 439–444.
27. Mitchell CK, Nguyen CK, Felman RM. Neuro-protection of retinal ganglion cells. Invest Ophthalmol Vis Sci 1998; 39: S261.
28. Serle JB. A comparison of the safety and efficacy of twice daily brimonidine 0.2% versus betaxolol 0.25% in subjects with elevated intraocular pressure. Surv Ophthalmol 1996; 41(suppl): S39–S47.
29. Littman L, Kempler P, Rhola M, *et al.* Severe symptomatic AV block induced by pilocarpine eye drops. Arch Intern Med 1987; 147: 586.
30. True-Gabelt B, Kaufman PL, Polanski JR. Ciliary muscle muscarinic binding sites, choline acetyltransferase and acetylcholinesterase in aging rhesus monkeys. Invest Ophthalmol Vis Sci 1990; 31: 24–31.
31. Strahlman ER, Vogel R, Tipping R, Cline-schmidt CM. The use of dorzolamide and pilocarpine as adjunctive therapy to timolol in patients with elevated intraocular pressure. The Dorzolamide Additivity Study Group. Ophthalmology 1996; 103: 1283–1293.
32. Silver LH. Clinical efficacy and safety of brinzolamide, a new topical carbonic anhydrase inhibitor for primary open-angle glaucoma and ocular hypertension. Am J Ophthalmol 1998; 126: 400–408.
33. Friedland BR, Mallonnee J, Anderson DR. Short-term dose response characteristics of acetazolamide in man. Arch Ophthalmol 1977; 95: 1809–1812.
34. Layton WM, Hallesy DM. Deformity of fore-limb in rats: association with high doses of acetazolamide. Science 1965; 149: 306–308.
35. Robbins R, Galin MA. Effect of osmotic agents on the vitreous body. Arch Ophthalmol 1969; 82: 694.

Chapter 17

Management protocols

Why should I read this chapter?

After all the reading you have done so far we finally get to the nitty gritty of how you actually manage the glaucoma patients you will be seeing day-in, day-out.

There is no simple algorithm which can be applied to the management of the glaucoma patient or the glaucoma suspect. Management should be tailored and individualized to each patient taking into account the patient's age, glaucoma status and their systemic status. It is reasonable to use generalized guidelines as a starting point, however each case must be considered in the context of the individual patient and their particular needs and characteristics.

Not all glaucoma patients require treatment. Over-treatment can cause significant problems. Patients may develop systemic side effects which may be potentially life threatening. There are also significant cost implications of lifelong treatment with glaucoma drops if treatment were not indicated.

Increasing use of prostaglandin analogs has led to an increase in prescribing rates and a rapid increase in cost.[1] At the same time, prescribing of beta-blockers has declined and trabeculectomy rates have fallen.

Much of the text so far has detailed the diagnostic challenge of making a definitive diagnosis of glaucoma. Hopefully at this stage we should have identified patients who are normal (and have thus been discharged from our care), glaucoma suspects, ocular hypertensives and those with definitive glaucoma.

Patients are entirely unique and exhibit different risk factors for disease, varying degrees of damage and subsequent rates of progression, contraindications to therapies, and other variables associated with their condition. It is the clinician's responsibility to take all these factors into account and devise a management strategy which is safe and efficacious for their patient.

Glaucoma suspects

Glaucoma suspects are not the same as ocular hypertensives. Ocular hypertensives have a risk factor for glaucoma (raised IOP) but have not developed any evidence of glaucomatous optic neuropathy, while glaucoma suspects are patients who cannot be confidently labeled as normal as they have features which may be consistent with glaucoma. The diversity of this group makes definitive or even rough guidance extremely difficult. If glaucoma suspects do turn out to have glaucoma then they are almost inevitably at a reasonably early stage of the disease as, if they had more significant evidence of damage, they would have been classified as glaucoma immediately.

The management of glaucoma suspects is highly case-specific. A decision has to be made in these patients as to whether they have glaucoma or not. If the decision is made that they now meet the criteria for glaucoma it needs to be determined whether they need treatment. Often such patients can be watched for change. There is usually time to play with. The clinical picture will evolve either in the form of development of features more consistent with glaucoma or definite stability of the condition, thereby lowering the suspicion of glaucoma and moving them closer to a possible discharge. Investigations using sensitive tests will assist in the differentiation of glaucoma from normal.

In some situations where the clear picture is not apparent but the clinical risks of missing a progressive glaucoma are too great, for example with an only eye, the patient may benefit from treatment even though the diagnosis is not clear cut. Naturally the risk versus benefit profile of the proposed treatment should be taken into account and a frank and open discussion with the patient should be undertaken before embarking upon treatment.

Ocular hypertensives

The OHT study has helped us understand which patients are in particular need of treatment. It has clearly shown that conversion to glaucoma is much more likely with higher pressures (no kidding!) and with thinner corneas (what we suspected anyway).

Patients with IOP repeatedly over 35 mmHg are at a greater than 50% risk of converting to glaucoma.[2,3] All patients regardless of age appear to be at at risk of developing a central retinal vein occlusion (CRVO) when they maintain a significantly raised IOP for an extended period.[4,5] CRVO is a disastrous ocular problem with significant visual morbidity; it is for this reason that the majority of clinicians tend to treat patients, regardless of CCT, with an IOP of above 30 mmHg, whether they have signs of glaucoma damage or not. The theory is that the high IOP causes compression of the venous system at the ONH, potentially facilitating stasis and the onset of a vein occlusion.

This arbitrary numerical IOP cut-off point goes against the ethos of not focusing too much on the pressure in isolation. A patient with an IOP of 28 mmHg and a CCT of 420 µm probably has a greater risk of developing a vein occlusion than a patient with an IOP of 30 mmHg and a CCT of 650 µm. Without any hard-and-fast evidence it is still the author's practice to treat OHT patients with an IOP of above 30 mmHg. Not only is this 30 mmHg cut-off point not validated but there is no definitive evidence to say that lowering IOP prevents the onset of vein occlusions. Patients with IOPs close to this threshold should have their CCT taken into consideration in the decision-making process.

OHT patients who are started on treatment probably do not require IOPs lower than 20 mmHg. Bringing them down to the upper limit of normal should hopefully prevent the onset of glaucoma damage.

Naturally deciding to treat or not to treat an OHT patient has to be done with consideration of the other ocular and patient factors. In patients with only one seeing eye the decision not to treat should be considered very carefully, as the risks of making the wrong clinical judgment are greater. Again the risk–benefit profile for treatment should be considered and the patient involved in the decision-making process.

Patients with ocular hypertension are at higher risk for developing glaucomatous visual field loss if their discs are suspect, if the IOP is higher and if the patient is older.[6] Ocular hypertensives who have pseudoexfoliation syndrome should be treated as they are at high risk of progressing to glaucoma.[7]

The newly diagnosed glaucoma patient

The decision has been made through clinical assessment, visual-field tests and ancillary investigations that the patient before you has glaucoma. Now you need to decide what to do with the patient. The majority of patients will need treatment, but not all. Making a diagnosis is good but it is also important to take other considerations into account before commencing treatment.

The aim of glaucoma management is to prevent the development of visual morbidity due to glaucoma in the patient's lifetime. In order to make a judgment on this we need to know the patient's likely survival. Of course this is impossible to know for sure, however an idea can be obtained from the patient's medical history and also from looking at the patient. Once we calculate a mental 'guesstimate' of the patient's likely lifetime we then need to know how quickly their glaucoma is progressing in order to make a judgment of whether they will experience ocular morbidity.

We do not always need to see progression to determine likely rate. If the patient already has glaucoma damage then we know that the worse the damage the more likely they are to progress, i.e. patients with a CDR of 0.9 are at real risk of getting worse. We can also look at the IOP to give us an idea of how quickly the patient is likely to deteriorate. We know that if the patient's IOP is 25–30 mmHg or even >30 mmHg the patient will get worse quickly. Conversely, if the IOP is 20 mmHg, the likely rate of progression will be slow in most (but not all) patients. Elderly patients with significant systemic comorbidity, mild to moderate glaucoma and a reasonably low IOP may be observed without treatment. Treatment can always be commenced at a later date if the clinical judgment was incorrect and the glaucoma progression exceeds the anticipated rate.

All treatment is aimed at reducing the IOP from the patient's baseline or presenting IOP. Hopefully the patient has had several IOP measurements to establish a realistic starting point. In an ideal world each patient would have a 24-hour diurnal IOP curve measured before treatment and then again after treatment. However in real clinical practice this is logistically impossible for most of us. Usually the IOP is measured in the morning (ideally) or the afternoon and as long as all subsequent IOP measurements post-treatment are at approximately the same time of day, a true idea of the IOP response to treatment can be elicited. Comparing morning pretreatment IOPs to an afternoon post-treatment IOP can give a false impression of efficacy as the patient's IOP may be lower anyway in the afternoon. All IOPs should have the time of measurement documented and the clinician should be aware of the potential effects of the diurnal variation.

In most cases, medical therapy is the first-line treatment. The choice of drop is dependent upon the individual patient but in the majority a prostaglandin analog is the drop of choice. In patients with a uveitic etiology for their glaucoma a prostaglandin analog is probably best avoided initially.

A target pressure (see Chapter 15) is set, based upon the presenting or baseline IOP, risk factors, patient characteristics and visual fields, and then treatment is instituted to achieve it.

In most patients a pressure reduction of more than 30% or to below 20 mmHg (whichever is the lower) is desirable. A drop should produce a more than a 10–15% reduction in IOP to be judged to be working adequately. If this pressure reduction is not achieved, and assuming the patient has been using the drops correctly, then the treatment is ineffective and should be stopped and another drop instituted. In some situations where the patient is on multiple therapy and we are still struggling to achieve target IOP, even an extra 5% IOP reduction may justify continued usage.

After starting treatment the patient should be seen approximately 4–6 weeks later to assess efficacy of the drop. This follow-up interval is of course dependent upon the individual patient's glaucoma status at diagnosis. In the presence of a markedly compromised optic nerve and a very high pressure the patient should be seen much sooner. It is inappropriate to leave a patient at risk of rapid glaucoma progression on a drop which may or may not be working. It should be made clear that patients should obtain repeat prescriptions from the general practitioner before they run out of drops.

At each follow-up visit, it is important to establish compliance and to determine whether the patient is experiencing any side effects or has any concerns about their treatment. If the desired target IOP is not achieved, then switching or adding medications should be contemplated.

In mild glaucoma visual fields should be repeated every 6 months for 2 years to obtain a baseline and understand the patient's long-term fluctuation. In moderate glaucoma it is reasonable to do visual fields every 4 months, and in advanced glaucoma fields may need to be done 3-monthly to ensure that there is no evidence of rapid progression.

The stable glaucoma patient

When a patient has had 18 months of follow-up, with achieved target pressures and stable optic nerve and visual-field parameters, the follow-up can be lengthened. IOP checks are usually scheduled every 6 months while visual-field assessments are usually carried out yearly. After several years of stability, follow-up may even be lengthened further depending upon the state of the individual patient.

Established progressing glaucoma patient

If progression of glaucoma has been documented by visual field or optic nerve comparisons, then compliance with medications must be assessed and optimized. If compliance has been good, then the target IOP has to be reset to a lower level and appropriate medical, laser or surgical therapy instituted to achieve it. IOP fluctuation must be considered as a possible causative factor and addressed appropriately by phasing. The new target pressure should usually be lowered by an additional 20–30%, depending upon the rate of this persistent progression.

Determining the effectiveness of medication

The prescribing of drops is not an innocuous undertaking. It is costly both in financial terms and in time. Time is invested by the patient every single day to use the drops. They also have to arrange for repeat prescriptions and make a special journey to collect their medications. They can suffer side effects, some of them obvious, such as allergy, and others that may lie hidden, such as impotence with beta-blocker use. If you are starting treatment on someone at the age of 40 they will be diligently using this for potentially the next 50 years. We need to ensure that they are on it because they are gaining benefit.

Different patients exhibit different responses to medications; some patients may respond better to beta-blockers than to a prostaglandin analog while others may respond better to alpha-agonists and not at all to a prostaglandin. The only way to determine this is by actually using the drop and assessing efficacy in each individual patient.

Monocular trials are the author's favored method for assessing efficacy. The main problem with treating only one eye and then seeing whether there is any effect is that adrenergic agents, such as beta-blockers and alpha-agonists, have crossover effects on the fellow eye.

Monocular trials take into account the patient's normal diurnal IOP curve and also control for interobserver variation in IOP measurement. We know that patients' IOPs can vary significantly between different clinic visits even if the readings are taken at the same time of day. By using the other eye as a control we can negate this variability.

A patient with an IOP of 26 mmHg in each eye may be commenced on treatment to both eyes. At their next clinic attendance their IOP is measured at 20 mmHg in the right eye and 21 mmHg in the left. Has there been any effect of the drop? It appears so, however we do not know whether the change simply represents the patient's normal IOP fluctuation over time. There is the potential that their IOP would have measured the same even had they not been on treatment. Had treatment been commenced in one eye only and the patient had come back with an IOP of 15 mmHg in the right and 21 mmHg in the left then there is proven efficacy (assuming that the treatment was indeed to the right eye!) and the treatment can now be started in the other eye. The response in one eye is usually strongly indicative of the response of the other eye.[8]

If the treatment was a beta-blocker or alpha-agonist then it is important to bear in mind that there will be an IOP-lowering effect on the opposite untreated eye, a phenomenon which muddies the water as regards efficacy.

Any changes in therapy necessitate another set of baseline IOP and visual-field measurements to form a standard to which evidence of further progression can be compared.

What drops to use?

The ideal drop to use is the one that reduces the IOP the best with the least adverse effects. This tends to be a prostaglandin analog. If there is no contraindication it makes sense to use prostaglandins as a first line treatment.

Which one? There are three main agents available and the literature would suggest that they are equally efficacious with very little difference between them. They are all well tolerated. Some may cause slightly more red eye than others but as a whole the choice of drop does not matter.

Assess efficacy to see if it is working. Have we achieved target IOP? If not then we need to decide to switch or add. If we have achieved a good IOP reduction in the first instance then adding makes sense.

What to add? Generally you have a choice of a beta-blocker, alpha-agonist, or carbonic anhydrase inhibitor (CAI). The author's preference is to try a beta-blocker next if there is no contraindication.

Again assess efficacy of the beta-blocker and be sure to question the patient about any potential side effects:

- Has your breathing been OK since the new drop has been started?
- Are you finding yourself out of puff?
- Do you feel light headed when you stand up?

It is worth laying a hand on the pulse to check the heart rate.

Are we at target IOP? If there has been no or minimal effect from the beta-blocker, discontinue it, i.e. switch to another drop rather than add. Generally it is not worth the long-term risks of beta-blocker use for only a 2–3 mmHg IOP reduction (although sometimes if we are struggling it is worth keeping them on this if we get to target IOP). If we have achieved a good IOP reduction but still not achieved target IOP we need to add another drop.

If beta-blockers are contraindicated or we are still not at target IOP then you have a choice of adding a CAI or alpha-agonist. Try them in your patients and see which one you prefer to move on to. The author tends to move on to a CAI to avoid the potential allergy problems seen with alpha-agonists.

Again assess efficacy and tolerability. At this stage the patient is usually on a prostaglandin analog and one or more of the remaining drops. Consider rationalizing their treatment and moving them over to combination drops. This should hopefully aid compliance but it also has cost implications. If you move to combination drops make sure you reassess efficacy. The combination drop may not work as well as the two separate drops in your patient. Remember that you are treating the unique individual in front of you and not the patients who were in the trials that reassured you of non-inferiority of the combination drops.

Possible combinations are:

- Prostaglandin + beta-blocker – use fixed combination prostaglandin and beta-blocker (e.g. Travatan, GanForte, Xalacom)
- Prostaglandin + beta-blocker + CAI – use fixed combination prostaglandin and beta-blocker (e.g. Travatan, GanForte, Xalacom) + CAI *or* use prostaglandin alone + fixed combination of beta-blocker and CAI (e.g. Cosopt)
- Prostaglandin + beta-blocker + alpha-agonist – use fixed combination prostaglandin and beta-blocker (e.g. Travatan, GanForte, Xalacom) + alpha-agonist *or* use prostaglandin alone + fixed combination of beta-blocker and alpha-agonist (e.g. Combigan)

Consider laser treatment in appropriate patients (see Chapter 18). There are no hard and fast rules as to when to embark upon laser treatment. Argon laser trabeculoplasty is infrequently used however the new selective laser trabeculoplasty seems to work well with a good safety profile. With the passage of time it will inevitably nudge its way into the standard hierachy of treatment for IOP reduction.

If despite our efforts we have not achieved target IOP medically then we need to consider surgical intervention.

References

1. Macleod SM, Clark R, Forrest J, Bain M, Bateman N, Azuara-Blanco A. A review of glaucoma treatment in Scotland 1994–2004. Eye 2006 Sep 22 (Epub ahead of print)

2. Pohjanpelto PEJ, Palva J. Ocular hypertension and glaucomatous optic nerve damage. Acta Ophthalmol 1974; 52: 194.
3. Kass MA, Hart WM Jr., Gordon M, *et al.* Risk factors favoring the development of glaucomatous visual field loss in ocular hypertension. Surv Ophthalmol 1980; 25: 155–162.
4. Luntz MH, Schenker HI. Retinal vascular accidents in glaucoma and ocular hypertension. Surv Ophthalmol 1980; 25: 163–167.
5. Chew EY, Trope GE, Mitchell BJ. Diurnal intraocular pressure in young adults with central retinal vein occlusion. Ophthalmology 1987; 94: 1545–1549.
6. Bengtsson B, Heijl A. A long-term prospective study of risk factors for glaucomatous visual field loss in patients with ocular hypertension. J Glaucoma 2005; 14: 135–138.
7. Grodum K, Heijl A, Bengtsson B. Risk of glaucoma in ocular hypertension with and without pseudoexfoliation. Ophthalmology 2005; 112: 386–390.
8. Realini T, Vickers WR. Symmetry of fellow-eye intraocular pressure responses to topical glaucoma medications. Ophthalmology 2005; 112: 599–602.

Chapter 18

Surgery and laser treatment for glaucoma

Why should I read this chapter?

The modern medications for glaucoma are highly effective and well tolerated. There will inevitably be patients, however, who do not achieve a low enough IOP on medication alone. There are others that will not tolerate the drops or not comply with the drops. How do we get the IOP down in this situation? We have a choice of laser trabeculoplasty or surgical intervention. This chapter is purposefully brief as most of this area is beyond the scope of this text. The shared care clinician needs to know when to refer to the glaucoma surgeon to consider laser or surgical intervention.

Laser trabeculoplasty

There are two forms of laser treatment in popular use for glaucoma. Historically argon laser trabeculoplasty (ALT) has been at the fore and indeed it was used in the Glaucoma Laser Trial (GLT). Recently a newer form of laser treatment has been developed called selective laser trabeculoplasty (SLT).

Argon laser trabeculoplasty

ALT was demonstrated in the GLT to be as effective as medications for the initial treatment of glaucoma.[1] It has been in use since the early 1980s and uses an argon laser of frequency 488–514 nm to photocoagulate the trabecular meshwork (TM) and improve aqueous outflow. Several theories have been suggested to explain the IOP-lowering effects of this laser treatment but definitive evidence is surprisingly lacking. The most widely accepted theories are the mechanical and cellular. According to the mechanical theory, ALT causes coagulative damage to the TM, which results in collagen shrinkage and scarring of the TM. This scarring and tightening at the site of each burn puts traction on the adjacent TM, opening adjacent intertrabecular spaces.[2-4] The cellular theory concentrates on the cellular response to these burns. Theoretically in response to the induced coagulative necrosis, there is migration of macrophages into the TM which then proceed to phagocytose and clear debris improving aqueous outflow and lowering IOP.

It is known, however, that the effectiveness of ALT decreases with time. ALT lowers the mean IOP by approximately 22% and may also reduce the incidence of diurnal IOP spikes in glaucoma patients.[5]

Elderly patients respond to ALT better than younger patients. ALT is more effective in POAG, pigmentary and pseudoexfoliative glaucomas and is less effective in uveitic, traumatic or steroid-induced glaucomas and in pseudophakic patients. ALT should not be attempted in patients with angle abnormalities such as narrow angles, peripheral anterior synechiae or angle neovascularization.

The decision to treat the entire 360° in one session or 180° in sequential sessions is subject to personal preference of the clinician. In one study, more IOP spikes were seen after treatment of a full 360° compared to 180°. However, not unexpectedly, the IOP-lowering effect was greater with 360° treatment.[6] When only half the angle is treated the other half can be treated at a second sitting if required. With pre- or post-treatment using apraclonidine or brimonidine, the occurrence of IOP spikes has been dramatically reduced.[7,8] Eventual loss of IOP control inevitably happens at some stage after ALT. Approximately 19% fail after 1 year, and an additional 10% fail each year thereafter, reaching a 65% failure rate at 5 years.[9] Once the whole angle is treated repeating the procedure is ineffective.[10] The clinical use of ALT is diminishing gradually.[11]

Selective laser trabeculoplasty

Different types of lasers with various wavelengths have been investigated for laser trabeculoplasty. Recently, a Q switched, frequency-doubled Nd:YAG laser using a frequency of 532 nm has been used for trabeculoplasty in glaucoma. In tissue cultures, it has been demonstrated that the low power and short duration of this laser can selectively target pigmented TM cells while sparing adjacent cells and tissues from collateral thermal damage, thus maintaining TM architecture.[12]

The exact mechanism of action of SLT is unknown. Since minimal mechanical damage is supposed to occur it would be logical to assume a cellular change to explain an improvement in aqueous outflow.

SLT uses a pulse duration of 3 ns compared with ALT which has a pulse duration in the range of 1 ms or greater. At pulse duration between 10 ns and 1 μs the energy is theoretically deposited within the target (pigmented TM cells) more rapidly than it can diffuse away, hence minimizing damage to the surrounding non-pigmented TM cells.[12]

The preliminary evidence on this treatment is quite encouraging.[13,14] Another benefit of SLT is that retreatment is possible whereas retreatment tends to be ineffective in ALT.

Cyclodiode laser

Cyclodestructive procedures aim to destroy part of ciliary body thus reducing aqueous inflow and reducing IOP. There are several different methods for achieving this but the one in most common use is the use of transscleral diode laser. Previously cyclodiode has been used solely for treatment in last ditch no-hope blind eyes. More and more it is being recognized that in appropriate controlled dosages it can be very effective in reducing IOP without compromising vision. Patients who have a painful blind eye with raised IOP (from for example rubeotic glaucoma) will definitely benefit from this laser as the risk from glaucoma surgery is not warranted and, moreover, surgery tends to carry a poor prognosis in these cases. Other cases of refractory glaucoma will likewise achieve reasonable pressure reduction with this technically straightforward treatment.

Titrating the iatrogenic ciliary body damage in small treatment doses will minimize the risk of inducing hypotony and ensuing phthisis bulbi. The smaller dosage will produce smaller stepwise IOP-lowering effects however the cost of this is that patients may require more than one treatment.

In patients with multiple previous failed glaucoma procedures, cyclodiode may be the intervention of choice even in well seeing eyes. Patients with a markedly raised IOP may have cyclodiode laser treatment to reduce their IOP as a temporizing measure before surgery can be undertaken.

Complications associated with cyclodiode procedures include conjunctival burns, anterior uveitis, loss of vision, pain, hyphema, vitreous hemorrhage, IOP spikes, hypotony, choroidal detachment, phthisis bulbi, malignant glaucoma, cataracts and, rarely but worryingly, sympathetic ophthalmitis.

Glaucoma filtering surgery

With improvement in surgical technique, adjunctive antifibrotic medications and vigilant postoperative care, the success rate of glaucoma filtering surgery in phakic primary open-angle glaucoma has improved to 80–90%. Complications, although rare, do occur and they can be potentially sight threatening.

Surgery should be considered when the patient fails to achieve their target IOP despite maximal medical therapy (MMT) or laser treatment. Potential clinical scenarios for consideration of surgical intervention:

- Signs of glaucoma progression at the lowest attainable IOP despite MMT.
- A degree of glaucoma damage which will (in the clinician's opinion) inevitably lead to glaucoma progression. For example, a 50-year-old patient with a CDR of 0.9 and a mean deviation of −25 dB who has an IOP of 25 mmHg despite MMT will almost inevitably progress and go blind in their lifetime. In such a scenario waiting for documented progression may be inappropriate and the patient should probably undergo surgery.
- Ocular hypertensive with IOP too high. Some OHT patients will have markedly raised IOPs despite MMT. In general if the IOP is above 30 mmHg despite MMT, surgery should be contemplated to lower IOP.
- Significant IOP fluctuation. Some patients on MMT may have a numerically good IOP at the lowest point of their diurnal curve but suffer significant fluctuation in IOP. Surgery will flatten the diurnal curve and prevent these spikes.[15]
- Poor compliance. Patients who do not comply with their medication may benefit from having surgery to lower IOP in the long term without the need for topical therapy. The patient will be required to use drops in the post-operative period and poor compliance in this critical period can have detrimental consequences not only on bleb survival but on vision as a whole.

Before surgical intervention is undertaken a frank and open discussion with the patient is required. They should be made aware of the intended procedure, the risks involved, the post-operative care which will be required and the ideal outcome. The need for post-operative manipulations and the importance of the use of post-operative medications should be emphasized.

The risks and benefits of the surgery should be contemplated. Are the benefits of surgery worth the risk? Consider the patient's rate of progression, their baseline glaucoma status (i.e. the severity of their glaucoma), their age and their circumstances. Will they suffer visual morbidity in their lifetime if you do not intervene to lower the IOP? If the answer is yes then surgery is indicated and they should be referred to the glaucoma surgeon.

Previously patients with an end-stage visual-field defect were not considered for surgery for fear of 'wipe-out'. There is a risk that glaucoma surgery itself may precipitate a stepwise progression of the patient's visual-field defect. In the setting of a small residual field this phenomenon could risk the patient's central vision, effectively wiping out what vision they have. Although this is still a risk which has to be explained and accepted by the patient it is actually a rare occurrence. In one study of 21 such cases there was no 'wipe-out'.[16]

One should also consider whether cyclodiode laser would be more appropriate than surgery (see above).

There are several different surgical techniques in use to lower IOP. At the forefront today are penetrating procedures in the form of trabeculectomy and non-penetrating procedures in the form of deep sclerectomy or viscocanalostomy. The precise surgical details and outcomes are beyond the scope of this text.

The management of the post-operative patient is highly specialized and would warrant a text in itself. Different surgeons you work with will have different protocols for their post-operative management. The aim is to achieve long-term IOP control with minimal complications.

In the setting of multiple failed glaucoma surgeries the insertion of a glaucoma drainage device may be appropriate. This is a highly specialized undertaking and is technically challenging. It involves the placement of a tube into the anterior chamber which takes aqueous out of the eye in a (hopefully) controlled fashion and facilitates drainage into the posterior subtenon space.

References

1. Glaucoma Laser Trial Research Group. The Glaucoma Laser Trial (GLT). Results of argon laser trabeculoplasty versus topical medicines. Ophthalmology 1990; 97: 1403–1413.
2. Reiss GR, Wilensky JT, Higginbotham EJ. Laser trabeculoplasty. Surv Ophthalmol 1991; 35: 407–428.
3. Wise JB, Witter SL. Argon laser therapy for open angle glaucoma. Arch Ophthalmol 1979; 97: 319–322.
4. Weinreb RN, Tsai CS. Laser trabeculoplasty. In: Ritch R, Shields MB, Krupin T, eds. The Glaucomas: Glaucoma Therapy, 2nd ed. Missouri: Mosby-Year Book, 1996; III: 1575–1590.
5. Greenidge KC, Spaeth GL, Fiol-Silva Z. Effect of argon laser trabeculoplasty on the glaucomatous diurnal curve. Ophthalmology 1983; 90: 800–804.
6. Honrubia FM, Ferrer EJ, Lecinena J, Torron C, Gomez ML. Long term follow-up of the argon laser trabeculoplasty in eyes treated 180 degrees and 360 degrees of the trabeculum. Int Ophthalmol 1992; 16: 375–379.

7. Threlkeld AB, Assalian AA, Allingham RR, *et al.* Apraclonidine 0.5% versus 1% for controlling intraocular pressure elevation after argon laser trabeculoplasty. Ophthalmic Surg Lasers 1996; 27: 657–660.
8. David R, Spaeth GL, Clevenger CE, *et al.* Brimonidine in the prevention of intraocular pressure elevation following argon laser trabeculoplasty. Arch Ophthalmol 1993; 111: 1387–1390.
9. Spaeth GL, Baez KA. Argon laser trabeculoplasty controls one third of cases of progressive, uncontrolled, open angle glaucoma for 5 years. Arch Ophthalmol 1992; 10: 491–494.
10. Richter CU, Shingleton BJ, Bellows AR, *et al.* Retreatment with argon laser trabeculoplasty. Ophthalmology 1987; 94: 1085–1089.
11. Albright CD, Schuman SG, Netland PA. Usage and cost of laser trabeculoplasty in the United States. Ophthalmic Surg Lasers 2002; 4: 334–336.
12. Latina MA, Park C. Selective targeting of trabecular meshwork cells: in vitro studies of pulsed and cw laser interactions. Exp Eye Res 1995; 60: 359–372.
13. Francis BA, Ianchulev T, Schofield JK, Minckler DS. Selective laser trabeculoplasty as a replacement for medical therapy in open-angle glaucoma. Am J Ophthalmol 2005; 140: 524–525.
14. Damji KF, Bovell AM, Hodge WG, *et al.* Selective laser trabeculoplasty versus argon laser trabeculoplasty: results from a 1-year randomised clinical trial. Br J Ophthalmol 2006; 90: 1490–1494.
15. Konstas AG, Topouzis F, Leliopoulou O, *et al.* 24-hour intraocular pressure control with maximum medical therapy compared with surgery in patients with advanced open-angle glaucoma. Ophthalmology 2006; 113: 765.e1.
16. Topouzis F, Tranos P, Koskosas A, *et al.* Risk of sudden visual loss following filtration surgery in end-stage glaucoma. Am J Ophthalmol 2005; 140: 661–666.

Chapter 19

Compliance

Why should I read this chapter?

Twenty percent of renal transplant patients do not take their medication, so how do we stand a chance as glaucoma specialists of getting our patients to take their drops in the hope of preventing worsening of a negative scotoma which, by definition, they don't even notice. We cannot always rely on our patients to take their prescribed medication. However sensible and cooperative they seem in front of you it is no guarantee that they will definitely use the drops you give them. They have other things going on in their lives and their glaucoma (whatever that is) isn't a priority. This chapter will hopefully help you maximize your chances of ensuring compliance.

Introduction

Chronic and, in particular, initially asymptomatic diseases, such as glaucoma, are susceptible to patient non-compliance to prescribed therapeutic regimens. The mainstay of glaucoma or OHT management is the reduction of IOP and this relies heavily on the use of medical therapy usually in the form of drops. We know these drops work and we can objectively quantify how much they are working by measuring a change in IOP. The drops tend to be quite well tolerated and administration usually takes less than a minute. And yet despite all this, non-adherence in patients with glaucoma is a major problem.

Patients with glaucoma do not get better, and they may get worse or even go blind despite our best efforts. Patients struggle to understand the need for preventative treatment particularly in conditions which do not have a high profile. High cholesterol is a demon which is frequently seen in the news and the link to heart disease is widely accepted. Patients can thus understand the need for cholesterol-lowering medication. They may not be so compliant with glaucoma therapy.

Patients expect some benefit from medication, either in the form of improved vision or improved ocular comfort. They do not achieve these with their glaucoma drops. When patients feel they do not benefit from a medication, they may ignore our instructions and not take their medication or take it infrequently.

Estimates of incidence

The exact magnitude of non-compliance in glaucoma will never be known precisely. Kass and colleagues[1-5] have found that 24% of patients on pilocarpine were non-compliant, whereas those on timolol were non-compliant in 18% of cases.[1,2] An interesting finding in this study was that the average patient on four times a day therapy instilled an average of only 2.6 drops per day.[1] Varying rates of non-compliance with glaucoma medication have been published ranging from 5–80%.[6-9]

A comprehensive study of aging and its effect on compliance showed that a large study population did not take prescribed therapy for 30% of the 12-month follow-up period.[10] Factors associated with non-adherence included the use of a glaucoma medication requiring more than two administrations per day and the presence of multiple other medications in the patient's drug regimen. An interesting finding of this study was that patients with more complex ocular medication schedules actually showed *greater* compliance, perhaps because the severity of their condition had been impressed on them more than it is on the average patient.

'One drop a night? How important can that be?'

Detecting non-compliance

The medical literature uses terms such as 'adherence' and 'compliance' interchangeably to describe the level of agreement between the prescribed treatment and actual patient practice. There are subtle differences but essentially they are the same issue. Recently 'persistency' has been utilized to describe adherence issues. It is defined as the total time on medical therapy and may be influenced by patient adherence, preference, efficacy and tolerability of the medication. It tends to refer to the situation in the United States whereby data on patient 'persistence' is elicited from the number of repeat prescriptions the patient submits. Healthcare issues whereby patients have to pay for their drops inevitably affect 'persistency'.

Adherence to prescribed treatment can be measured by either direct or indirect methods. Direct methods include observation, measurement of drug concentrations in blood or urine and detection of biological markers of efficacy. Indirect methods include patient questionnaires and diaries, rates of repeat prescription presentation and measurement of physiological markers of compliance (such as IOP reduction). Each method has its own advantages and disadvantages.

Electronic monitoring systems (an indirect method) have provided detailed information about patterns of patient behavior in taking glaucoma medications. Most non-compliance occurs with dose omissions (rather than extra dose application) or delays in the timing of dosages.[11,12] A large systematic review of 76 trials in which electronic monitors were used for a variety of medical therapies concluded that patient adherence to medications was inversely proportional to frequency of dosing.[13] Moreover, patients generally improve their compliance just before their doctor's appointment, a phenomenon that has been called the 'white-coat adherence'.

Studies using electronic monitors of compliance have documented six general patterns of medication adherence in patients treated for chronic illnesses.[14] Patient behavior falls into six categories with a sixth of the patient population fitting into each category:

(1) Nearly perfect adherence to a regimen
(2) Takes nearly all the prescribed doses, but with some timing irregularity
(3) Miss an occasional single day's dose and have timing inconsistency
(4) Take drug holidays three or four times a year, with occasional omissions of doses

(5) Have a drug holiday monthly or more often, with frequent omissions

(6) Take few or no doses while giving the impression of adequate adherence[15]

In order to change patient compliance we need to understand why our patients do not comply with their treatment so that we can devise methods to intervene. Barriers to compliance have recently been described for patients with glaucoma.[16]

Structured interviews were carried out with 48 glaucoma patients eliciting 71 obstacles to compliance. These obstacles were grouped into four separate categories: situational/environmental factors (49%), medication regimen factors (32%), patient-related factors (16%) and provider-related factors (3%). The aforementioned study was carried out in the US and patients included in this study were a select group who had health insurance and thus their attitudes to their glaucoma medication may have been skewed.

It is clear from the various studies published that doctors are very poor at picking out which of their patients are non-compliant. So how do we know if our patients are complying with their medication or not?

Realistically asking the patient is the most practical way we can assess compliance in a clinical setting. Kass and colleagues interviewed 141 patients and reported that they admitted to missing only 3% of drop administrations.[5] From the data above we can see that this appears too good to be true and probably indicates that even when formally interviewed patients do not acknowledge their missed treatments.

Although it is impossible to be certain about compliance, certain interviewing skills and techniques may assist in determining how close a patient is getting to their prescribed regimen. Open-ended questions such as 'what drops do we have you on at the moment?' will elicit much more than a simple 'are you using your drops?' to which a quick 'yes' will be forthcoming. Taking a few moments to question spouses or carers will also glean valuable information.

Clinical effect is a key method for detecting compliance. After all, this is why we are concerned about compliance. The patient has glaucoma and we treat them with drops. Intuitively we know that should they not use their drops they will worsen. Thorough and methodical clinical assessment of morphology and functional change at each follow-up is vital. A patient progressing despite an apparent 'target' IOP at clinic follow-up should immediately raise concerns that the patient is not complying. Being open and honest with the patient about your suspicions and concerns can allow them to divulge the truth about their actual compliance with medication.

Some of the medications we use have distinct secondary effects such as miosis with pilocarpine or lash and/or iris pigmentation with prostaglandin analogs. These may be used as surrogate markers for compliance.

Why do patients not comply?

There are several reasons possible for non-compliance and often there is a combination of factors at play. The causology profile for non-compliance will inevitably vary with regard to certain patient characteristics. For example reasons for non-compliance may be very different for an 80-year old man who lives alone compared to a 30-year old businessman with a busy family life.

Some of the most common causes of non-compliance are:

1. Side effects (ocular and systemic)
2. Frequency/inconvenience of instillation
3. Lack of adequate understanding of disease and medication instructions

4. Polypharmacy
5. Miscellaneous factors

Side effects

Many patients complain of bothersome ocular side effects of topical glaucoma medications, the most common being stinging and redness. Dry-eye patients may experience worsening of their symptoms once glaucoma drops are added and their already compromised corneas are pickled in preservatives. The presence of any ocular side effects when using a drop which has no immediate identifiable benefit to the patient will inevitably lead them to question the need for the treatment.

Systemic absorption of topical glaucoma medications can result in a variety of side effects (see Chapter 16).

It is important to continually reinforce the reasons for taking glaucoma medications at each and every clinical visit. Often forewarning the patient about potential minor side effects may help them expect them and may facilitate a level of acceptance.

Patients should be actively questioned about side effects, the presence of which do not necessarily mean that that drug should be immediately discontinued. Any adverse side effects should be balanced against the efficacy of the drop. Minor self-limiting stinging or a bad taste in the mouth may be accepted if the effect of the drop is dramatic. The patient should be actively engaged in any decision to continue such a drop and this formal agreement will help cement their compliance.

At every review the patient should be informed regarding their glaucoma status in whichever fashion is most appropriate to that patient. It should be emphasized that they have not worsened because of the drops and that should the drops be stopped they will deteriorate.

Frequency/inconvenience of instillation

There is no doubt that drops are inconvenient to use. The patient needs to carry them with them when they are away. They need to remember when to put them in every single day of their lives regardless of what other life issues are occurring. Every month they need to submit a repeat prescription request to get more of their medication and somehow arrange to collect it. It is important to emphasize that the benefits of the drops outweigh the inconvenience of using them.

Frequency of instillation may also have an impact on compliance. In patients in whom drop instillation is difficult for whatever reason, a once-daily medication may be preferable to a twice-daily dose. In one UK-based study patients treated with a once-daily prostaglandin analog demonstrated lower rates of therapy failure and therapy discontinuation compared with patients treated with other widely used IOP-lowering medications, including beta-blockers.[17] There is further evidence that prostaglandins are associated with better persistence and adherence than any other drug class.[18] Another study showed an average of 76% adherence with prostaglandin analogs so even using once-daily drops does not ensure full compliance.[19] Naturally, other factors such as the side-effect profile of the drop may play a role in these findings.

One potential disadvantage to once-daily dosing is that patients are less likely to miss both instillations of a twice-daily medication meaning that they get IOP lowering for at least half of that day, while if they miss their once-daily drug they risk a high IOP for a whole 24-hour period.

The need to adhere to a delay between drop instillation to avoid washout when using multiple drops can be a problem and a potential argument for the use of combination drops to aid compliance. Washout of drops is a well established phenomenon.[20] It has been shown that leaving only a 30 second delay between drop administrations leads to 45% of drug loss. Leaving 2 minutes between doses leads to 17% drug loss and by 5 minutes there is no loss of drug. All patients should be told to leave at least 5 minutes between drops to prevent washout and loss of efficacy. If a patient uses three drops on a twice daily basis then they have to spend 15 minutes each time they apply their drops. Patients may begrudge giving 30 minutes of their day over to drop administration unless they understand (and accept) the need for treatment. Clearly combination drops will have a role to play to minimize this amount of time and hopefully aid compliance.

Lack of understanding

Unsurprisingly, poor patient understanding of their disease and the need for the treatment they are on, has a negative impact upon compliance.

The visit when glaucoma is first diagnosed is a keystone in engaging the patient in their disease. The clinician needs to take a bit of time to explain the disorder clearly and explain the nature of the visual loss caused by glaucoma. A fine balance has to be struck between scaring the patient with stories of how they 'will permanently and irreversibly lose patches of their peripheral vision if they do not comply with their drops' and being so reassuring that you do not emphasize the severity of the disorder you will be treating for them for the rest of their lives. The level to which you have to instill fear depends upon the individual patient. If compliance is impossible without scaring the patient then scare them but do it cautiously and considerately. Causing undue anxiety in a patient who would have complied with treatment anyway is unnecessary and may actually cause significant psychological morbidity. Do no harm.

Education regarding drop dosages and timing, as well as instillation technique is also of critical importance. Kass and colleagues found that only 20% of patients in their study reported being instructed on how to instill their drops.[5]

Miscellaneous

Other factors that have been implicated as reasons for non-compliance are increasing age,[21] gender (male patients have been shown to be less compliant),[22] race and increased time in the waiting room.[23] Furthermore, patients with definitely diagnosed glaucoma may be more likely to adhere to therapy than patients who are only glaucoma suspects,[18] presumably because they perceive the benefit of treatment when they have established damage and a definite diagnosis.

Patients who dislike their physicians also tend to be less compliant, emphasizing the need to generate a rapport with our patients. Not only are they more likely to comply but they will also return to see you, keeping you in a job.

Increasing compliance

So how do we increase compliance?

Educating the patient is the key. Educating a patient takes time, but that time is an essential investment on the part of the treating clinician. Once the patient is hooked early on and their drop regimen enters their everyday life routine then the chance for achieving long-term compliance is enhanced.

As clinicians we have several opportunities for intervention to make a difference in our patient's clinical course and potentially to thereby alter the prognosis.

First visit

The initial clinic visit is a crucial time for setting the stage for long-term compliance. Whenever patients attend us for the first time we have to either formally or subconsciously enter into a 'care agreement' or 'contract of care' with them. We undertake to do our best for them and ensure the preservation of their visual function and they in turn agree to attend the clinic appointments and undergo any investigations and treatments we see fit. With glaucoma this is a contract which is binding for the rest of their lives and often for the rest of your professional life. It is not something to launch into lightly and it should be made clear to the patient at the outset what their side of the bargain will be. In the event of poor compliance the clinician can rightfully refer back to the original agreement and question why they did not do what they said they would.

In order to cement this bond between patient and clinician it is important that a rapport is developed at an early stage. Take time to impress in clear, succinct and appropriate language the significance of their disease and the ways in which we will aim to tackle their problem and prevent visual loss. Visual aids can be helpful in explaining the condition and the response to treatment.

A discussion of how treatment prevents visual loss by lowering the pressure in the eye should also be undertaken, with emphasis that lowering IOP will not be felt by the patient, but will be measured by the clinician.

Literature

Provision of literature explaining their condition and the need for treatment can be invaluable. Patients may be overwhelmed in the clinic and not take in everything you tell them. Giving them the chance to reflect upon the condition by reading a clear and pointed text in the comfort of their own home can improve understanding.

Written instructions with regards their drop regimen is invaluable and has been shown to be good for compliance.[24] Patients on complicated regimens should be offered treatment charts with the times of their drops clearly presented.

Carers

Getting carers on side can be an excellent asset in the fight for compliance. Family members should be involved in the initial discussion of the disease and also at each subsequent visit. If they become involved in the patient's care from the outset they can help enforce the need for compliance and also objectively (and hopefully honestly) report any lack of compliance.

Subsequent visits

Patients may attend you only twice or in some situations only once in a year. Each visit should be seen as an opportunity not only to confirm compliance but also to reinforce and re-emphasize the need for compliance. Questioning the patients and their carers/family members directly about their adherence to medication will highlight any discrepancies.

Involve the patient in their target IOP. Tell them what you are aiming for and they will gradually begin to ask at each visit what their IOP is. The link between their drop usage and the consistently good IOP seen in the clinic should be made clear and hopefully some conditioning towards compliance will begin to form. This must be used with caution as patients may become overly anxious about a reading a few mmHg out of their ideal range even though this is clinically not significant.

Ancillary staff

You are not alone in managing your glaucoma patient. There will inevitably be other staff available who will help you in educating and caring for your patient. Nurses and other health workers can be a valuable asset in explaining glaucoma to the patient and their families. Sometimes patients feel anxious when faced with the doctor and do not open up fully and ask the questions they truly wished to ask. Speaking to other staff can help break down those barriers. However, we still need to recognize these barriers within ourselves and seek to change our practice so that we gain the patient's trust.

Proper drop instillation technique should be taught on the first visit, with supplementary training at follow-up visits. Patients' drop technique should be assessed regularly to ensure the drop is actually getting into the eye. This can highlight numerous problems, including problems squeezing the bottle, an issue common with elderly arthritic patients.

Digital nasolacrimal occlusion (i.e. pressure over the nasolacrimal sac after drop installation) should be encouraged as this technique enhances drug delivery to the eye and minimizes systemic absorption and thus bothersome side effects.

Communication

This is really the key. We need to communicate effectively with our patients to ensure they know their disorder and know the benefits of their treatment. Communication is not simply a matter of verbalizing the facts. There is much more to it. It should be tailored to the individual. For example the explanation of their glaucoma offered to an experienced nurse will be different to the one utilized for a 25-year-old laborer. The facts remain the same but the way in which they are communicated can be vastly different.

We have to foster faith in us and our abilities so that our patients trust us. When treating patients it is important the possible adverse ocular and systemic side effects of the drugs are discussed. If a patient experiences something they were warned about they will be more accepting of it. If it comes as a surprise because the clinician made no mention of it they will lose confidence.

Instructions should be given to contact the glaucoma service if they run into problems with the drops, rather than stop them for an extended period of time until their next follow-up. Discuss with them what to do if they accidentally miss a dosage. Explain that they should put the drop in as soon as they remember, and then simply get back on their original regimen. The patient should be asked to bring the drops with them on each follow-up visit, and occasionally asked to describe and demonstrate how the drops are used. This gives the practitioner a better sense of compliance than simply assuming that instructions are being followed.

Tell the patient when you commence treatment that it is a long-term treatment and that although they are given a prescription for 28 days of drops they will need to attend their general practitioner for repeat prescriptions. If they stop treatment after just 1 month, not only will their IOP be raised again until their next follow-up, but that follow-up will be a wasted visit as they will again be untreated and the only course of action will be to re-prescribe them medication.

Social status and education

There is no clear link between social status/education and adherence. We are failing our patients if we presume that a cause for their poor compliance is poor education or low social status. The link is between patient education and compliance. Patients in a lower social class may or may not have a poor level of education. They may need different approaches to the education regarding their glaucoma. They may need more time. They may need the condition explained in different terms. They may need more aggressive descriptions to convince them of their need to comply with treatment and reattend. They may have to listen to accounts of how they will lose their driving licence and thus lose their job if they do not comply with treatment and follow-up. Each case is specific and there is no 'one-size-fits-all' answer to patient education. We are doing our patient a disservice if we do not spend the time actively to get them to a level of understanding whereby they are likely to comply.

Non-compliant patients

Despite all of our best efforts some patients do not comply with the medical regimen prescribed or do not bother turning up for their appointments. We can only do so much and all of the strategies above may still fail. Involving the patient's general practitioner is an important step as they may have insight into why the patient is not attending or not using their medication.

Some patients with poor compliance should be considered for laser or surgical therapy. Patients undergoing surgery will need drops post-operatively as well as an intensive follow-up regimen. If the patient is a poor complier they may not use their drops, causing a technically successful procedure to fail. Of even more concern is the fact that if a patient does not reattend after surgery they can run into potentially blinding complications.

Conclusion

Some patients will comply with treatment whether you do a good job of ensuring it or not. There are others where it will take time and effort. Taking this time and effort is a vital part of caring for glaucoma patients. Their condition is life-long and they may be at risk of eventual blindness despite everything we do for them. We need to continually ensure our patients are complying with the treatment we give them and use every trick in the book to spot those who aren't and somehow change them.

References

1. Kass MA, Meltzer DW, Gordon M, *et al*. Compliance with topical pilocarpine treatment. Am J Ophthalmol 1986; 101: 515.
2. Kass MA, Gordon M, Morley RE Jr, *et al*. Compliance with topical timolol treatment. Am J Ophthalmol 1987; 103: 188.
3. Kass MA, Hodapp E, Gordon M, *et al*. Part I. Patient administration of eyedrops: interview. Ann Ophthalmol 1982; 14: 775.
4. Kass MA, Meltzer DW, Gordon MO. A miniature compliance monitor for eyedrop medication. Arch Ophthalmol 1984; 102: 1550.
5. Kass MA, Hodapp E, Gordon M, *et al*. Part II. Patient administration of eyedrops: observation. Ann Ophthalmol 1982; 14: 889.
6. Olthoff CM, Schouten JS, van de Borne BW, Webers CA. Noncompliance with ocular hypotensive treatment in patients with glaucoma or ocular hypertension an evidence-based review. Ophthalmology 2005; 112: 953–961.
7. Rotchford AP, Murphy KM. Compliance with timolol treatment in glaucoma. Eye 1998; 12: 234–236.
8. Gurwitz JH, Glynn RJ, Monane M, *et al*. Treatment for glaucoma; adherence for the elderly. Am J Public Health 1993; 83: 711–716.
9. Patel SC, Spaeth GL. Compliance in patients prescribed eyedrops for glaucoma. Ophthalmic Surg 1995; 26: 233–236.
10. Chang JS Jr, Lee DA, Petursson G, *et al*. The effect of a glaucoma medication reminder cap on patient compliance and intraocular pressure. J Ocular Pharmacol 1991; 7: 117.
11. Burnier M. Long-term compliance with antihypertensive therapy: another facet of chronotherapeutics in hypertension. Blood Press Monit 2000; 5 (Suppl 1); S31–S34.
12. Paes AH, Bakker A, Soe-Agnie CJ. Impact of dosage frequency on patient compliance. Diabetes Care 1997; 20: 1512–1517.
13. Claxton AJ, Cramer J, Pierce C. A systematic review of the associations between dose regimens and medication compliance. Clin Ther 2001; 23: 1296–1310.
14. Osterberg L, Blaschke T. Adherence to medication. N Engl J Med 2005; 353: 487–497.
15. Fingeret M, Schuettenberg SP. Patient drug schedules and compliance. J Am Optom Assoc 1991; 62: 478–480.
16. Tsai JC, McClure CA, Ramos SE, Schlundt DG, Pichert JW. Compliance barriers in glaucoma: a systematic classification. J Glaucoma 2003; 12: 393–398.
17. Zhou Z, Althin R, Sforzolini BS, Dhawan R. Persistency and treatment failure in newly diagnosed open angle glaucoma patients in the United Kingdom. Br J Ophthalmol 2004; 88: 1391–1394.
18. Nordstrom BL, Friedman DS, Mozaffari E, Quigley HA, Walker AM. Persistence and adherence with topical glaucoma therapy. Am J Ophthalmol 2005; 140: 598–606.
19. Wilensky J, Fiscella RG, Carlson AM, *et al*. Measurement of persistence and adherence to regimens of IOP-lowering glaucoma medications using pharmacy claims data. Am J Ophthalmol 2006; 141 (1 Suppl): S28–33.

20. Eriksen SP, Robinson JR, Chrai SS, Makoid MC. Drop size and initial dosing frequency problems of topically applied ophthalmic drugs. J Pharm Sci 1974; 63(3): 333–338.
21. Gurwitz JH, Glynn RJ, Monane M, *et al.* Treatment for glaucoma: adherence by the elderly. Am J Pub Health 1993; 83: 711–716.
22. Bloch S, Rosenthal AR, Friedman L, *et al.* Patient compliance in glaucoma. Br J Ophthalmol 1977; 61: 531.
23. Kass MA. Non-compliance to ocular therapy. Glaucoma reports. Ann Ophthalmol 1978; 10: 1244.
24. Kharod BV, Johnson PB, Nesti HA, Rhee DJ. Effect of written instructions on accuracy of self-reporting medication regimen in glaucoma patients. J Glaucoma 2006; 15: 244–247.

Section 4

Specific Glaucoma Entities

Glaucoma is not a single entity. It is important to understand that there are many different varieties of this condition, all of which end up at a common pathological end-point of glaucomatous optic neuropathy. Detecting these conditions and comprehension of how the management of them may vary from the 'ordinary' open-angle glaucoma is vital.

Chapter 20

Normal-tension glaucoma

Normal-tension glaucoma (NTG) is a reasonably common diagnosis. Even the studies which were specifically designed to examine this disease entity used different criteria for making the diagnosis. Some glaucoma specialists believe that it is simply one end of a pressure-related disease spectrum and not a separate disease entity in its own right. NTG is certainly similar to its big brother POAG in many ways, however it is also different in several key features, the most obvious of which is the lack of raised IOP.

Since its first description by von Graefe in 1857[1], various definitions of normal-tension glaucoma have been suggested and widely used. A 1998 survey of 63 articles pertaining to NTG published between 1973 and 1997 revealed that the range of maximum IOP levels acceptable for categorization of NTG was broad, from 17 mmHg to 26 mmHg.[2] In more than 40% of these studies, including the Collaborative Normal-Tension Glaucoma Study Group, patients with IOP higher than 21 mmHg were acceptable for study inclusion.

A sensible definition of *normal*-tension glaucoma is that the IOP is normal, i.e. within 2 standard deviations of the mean, the angles are open, and that there are features of the optic nerve and visual field which are consistent with glaucomatous optic neuropathy. Thus an IOP of less than 21 mmHg seems a good way to define NTG.

An IOP consistently less than 21 mmHg at the morning clinic is not enough to make a diagnosis. We need to have an accurate measure of the patient's diurnal IOP curve before we can make this diagnosis. All patients should have IOP phasing before a confident diagnosis of NTG can be made.

We as clinicians need to be sensible about this diagnosis. We need to ask ourselves the question 'so what?' Does it make a difference if I label this patient as NTG or POAG? Will my management be different? In the great majority of cases the answer is no. There are certain clinical situations whereby the patient will be managed differently and their prognosis may diverge from that of a high-pressure glaucoma patient.

Take two patients both with IOPs of 20 mmHg in the morning. Both have appearances consistent with glaucoma. Both are phased and one is found to have an IOP which goes up to 23 mmHg at 6 pm while in the other the IOP goes up to 21 mmHg. One is labeled an NTG patient while the other is a POAG. Does this difference in labeling have true clinical significance? Will these patients have a different clinical course and should they have different management? Well, probably not. Granted one patient has an IOP fluctuation of 3 mmHg while the other has less of a fluctuation but in terms of NTG versus POAG the distinction is probably not required.

In both you will treat them with IOP-lowering medication as they probably have pressure-dependent disease. Take corneal thickness into account as well and it will mean that the arbitrary classification based on one IOP cut-off point is meaningless. The patient above with an IOP peaking at 21 mmHg may have a corneal thickness of 450 μm compared to the patient peaking at 23 mmHg who may have a corneal thickness of 600 μm.

Phasing becomes important when the IOPs are towards the middle to bottom of the normal range. Take two patients with IOPs of 12 mmHg at their morning clinic attendances and a suspicion of glaucoma. Phasing reveals that one has a steady IOP of 12 mmHg throughout the day while the other has an IOP which fluctuates and peaks at 21 mmHg. The latter probably has pressure-dependent disease and will more than likely behave as a POAG. The former with an IOP of 12 mmHg consistently is the one we are interested in and the one with true 'normal-tension glaucoma'. This patient probably does not have pressure-dependent disease or maybe they have only partially pressure-dependent pathology. This is an important thing to recognize when everything we do to the patient is normally designed to bring IOP down. In such patients we need to look for other pathologies (such as compressive lesions) or consider vascular or vasospastic disorders as playing a part.

Epidemiology

There is a wide discrepancy in the published literature regarding the prevalence of NTG because no consistent and reproducible definition of the disease is used. NTG is now known to be a common form of glaucoma.[3] NTG probably accounts for approximately 25–30%[4,5] of all glaucoma cases, but there is probably a significant amount of under-detection.

In the Baltimore Eye Survey[6] 16.7% of glaucomatous eyes never had a recorded IOP exceeding 21 mmHg and thus matched our definition for NTG.

Gender

The gender predeliction, if any, of NTG is controversial and disputed. Many studies suggest that women are at greater risk of developing NTG while others suggest no such link.[7] There is some evidence[8] suggesting that men are more severely affected in the early stages of the disease, while women have an overall worse prognosis.[9]

Pathophysiology of normal-tension glaucoma

Role of blood flow

The principal arterial blood supply to the anterior optic nerve is via the short posterior ciliary arteries. The prelaminar and laminar region of the anterior optic nerve is supplied by direct branches of these vessels and by vessels originating from the arterial circle of Zinn-Haller. The retrolaminar region is primarily supplied by branches of the pial arteries and the short posterior ciliary arterial system. The blood supply to the nerve is very complex, and marked variation is seen between individuals. The intricate and incompletely understood nature of the vascular supply to the ONH may explain why we have not fully elucidated the true cause of NTG.

Various factors affect blood flow to the ONH, including vasospastic tendencies, local auto-regulation mechanisms, IOP, blood viscosity, perfusion pressure, venous drainage and the normal variation in the nature of blood supply to the ONH.

The vasculature and blood flow of the ONH in patients with NTG differs from that of patients with POAG and non-glaucomatous patients. Systolic and diastolic blood flow velocities of the retrobulbar vessels in NTG, POAG and controls have been measured. A significant increase in vascular resistance and a decrease in blood flow velocity (especially end-diastolic velocity) is seen in the ophthalmic artery, central retinal artery and posterior ciliary arteries of patients with NTG or POAG when compared to control patients.[10–13] Experimentally increasing IOP has no effect on the ophthalmic and posterior ciliary artery perfusion suggesting to researchers that other factors are probably responsible for the vascular pathogenesis of NTG.[13–15]

There is increasing evidence that systemic vascular dysregulation and localized vasospasm are factors in the pathogenesis of NTG.[16–18]

Role of nocturnal blood pressure

Nocturnal hypotension, either normal (physiological) or secondary (for example due to antihypertensive medication), may reduce flow of blood to the ONH, potentially resulting in ischemia.[19] This nocturnal blood pressure dip appears to be significantly greater in NTG patients than in POAG and controls and has been implicated as a potential causative or contributory factor.[20–23] Nocturnal blood pressure parameters tend to be even lower in glaucoma patients with progressive visual-field defects compared with patients who were stable.[24]

One study[25] assessed a series of NTG patients and found that a third were 'non-dippers', while two thirds has evidence of significant or marked nocturnal blood pressure dipping. They theorized that these blood pressure fluctuations could potentially affect the mean ocular perfusion pressure and compromise ONH blood flow and predispose to NTG.

Role of CCT

Evidence exists that patients with NTG have significantly thinner central corneas ($521 \pm 31\,\mu m$) when compared with controls ($555 \pm 34\,\mu m$) and patients with POAG ($556 \pm 35\,\mu m$).[26,27] By applying corrective nomograms for CCT,[28] we may be underestimating the IOP in NTG patients by an average of 2.3 mm Hg.[29] In one study,[26] when corneal thickness was taken into account, 31% of the NTG patients met the diagnostic criteria for POAG.

Role of intraocular pressure

The role of the IOP in the pathogenesis of NTG is still not fully understood. One study demonstrated that in 12 of 14 cases of NTG with asymmetric IOP, the NTG was worse in the eye with the higher IOP.[30] This suggests that IOP does play some role in the disease.

Another study[31] studied 23 bilateral but asymmetric cases of NTG and showed that 12 patients had more severe visual field loss in the eye with the higher IOP, but 11 had more severe loss in the eye with the lower IOP.

In a population of 59 NTG patients[32] 47 patients had asymmetric visual-field defects, but only 13 of these also had asymmetric IOP. In most cases, the eye with the higher IOP had the more pronounced visual-field loss, but the majority of patients with asymmetric visual-field loss had an equal IOP in each eye. This data seems to suggest that IOP is not the most important pathogenetic factor in NTG.

There is also some evidence to suggest the IOP fluctuation also plays a role in risk of glaucoma progression in NTG patients.[33,34]

Results of the research are clearly conflicting, however it is clear that IOP does play a role in some patients with NTG. The magnitude of this role varies considerably between different groups of patients.

Role of IOP reduction

In the late 1990s, evidence showed that lowering IOP, both surgically[35] and medically,[36] probably slows the rate of progression of NTG. In a study of 17 patients with progressive bilateral NTG, each received a unilateral trabeculectomy while the other eye was untreated and was used as a control.[35] The rate of visual-field loss progression was significantly less in the treated eye.

The Collaborative Normal-Tension Glaucoma Study Group was a large multicenter, prospective, randomized, controlled clinical trial which provided evidence that IOP reduction was effective in NTG (see Chapter 25).[36]

Optic nerve head morphology

As with all glaucomas there is no hard-and-fast rule with regard to the appearance of the optic nerve head. Some characteristics of the optic nerve of patients with NTG appear to present with greater frequency when compared with non-glaucomatous eyes or the optic nerve of patients with POAG.

Size of the optic nerve head and neuroretinal rim

There is evidence to suggest that mean optic disc area is larger in patients with NTG than in patients with POAG.[37,38] NTG discs also tend to have thinner neuroretinal rim tissue located in the inferior and inferior temporal quadrants.[36]

Acquired pits of the optic nerve

Acquired pits of the optic nerve are discrete, focal areas of excavation within the lamina cribrosa at the base of the optic cup (Fig. 7.9). They may represent a structural weakness of the lamina cribrosa or a localized area of ischemic damage.[36] Pits were reported by one study[39] to occur in 74% of a population with NTG and in 15% of a population with POAG. They are usually located in the inferior quadrant (70%) or the superior quadrant (30%) of the cup.[40] Unsurprisingly dense visual-field defects with steep borders correlate with the location of pits.

Optic disc hemorrhages

The reported prevalence of ODHs in NTG varies from 10–64%.[41–43] Disc hemorrhages are more frequently seen in NTG rather than in POAG.[44–46] They can also represent an early sign of glaucoma damage and may precede the onset of visual-field loss.[47]

Retinal nerve fiber layer defects

Localized (slit or wedge) NFL defects, as opposed to diffuse NFL loss, have been reported to occur more commonly in NTG than in POAG.[48,49]

Peripapillary atrophy

PPA appears more commonly in NTG than POAG.[50] We do not know why PPA occurs but there are theories that it is a manifestation of vascular ischemia to the choroidal circulation which would fit nicely with a vascular insufficiency story for NTG.

Visual field loss

Patients with NTG have glaucomatous visual-field defects which are often completely indistinguishable from their high-pressure counterparts. There are a few features which tend to be more often seen in NTG rather than POAG. The field loss in NTG tends to show more localized defects,[51,52] a steeper slope of the defect,[53,54] and a defect closer to central fixation (Fig. 11.5).[55]

Treatment

The Collaborative Normal-Tension Glaucoma Study (CNTGS) showed that lowering IOP by 30% significantly reduced the rate of progression in patients with NTG. In this landmark study, beta-blockers and adrenergic drugs were not used because of theoretical concerns of ONH blood supply compromise. The hierachy of treatment was pilocarpine, laser trabeculoplasty and filtering surgery to achieve a 30% reduction from the baseline IOP. Other drops were not available at the start of the trial and thus they were not used to achieve this 30% IOP reduction. It should also be noted that patients recruited into the CNTGS had quite marked optic neuropathy and so taking the findings to be gospel for early NTG may potentially be erroneous.

   The fact that two thirds of patients in the control arm did not progress despite no treatment makes us wonder whether it is worth treating NTG patients at all. Some clinicians advocate watching for progression before initiating treatment. If the severity of the field loss is relatively minimal and the patient can do reliable visual fields then this seems to be a sensible option. It avoids targeting the two thirds of patients who would not have progressed anyway.

Arguing against this is the fact that we know patients with NTG tend to have field defects which are closer to fixation and that are deeper and steeper in nature. Awaiting manifest progression may result in irreversible central field loss, although in clinical practice this does not seem to occur. Targeting patients with field defects very close to fixation for treatment, even without documented progression, seems to be prudent.

Each patient has to be treated on an individual case-by-case basis. If the benefits of treatment outweigh the risks, then treatment should be offered.

Beta-blockers tend to have little effect on IOP in NTG and may have theoretical adverse effects on ONH blood flow. It may be that because aqueous outflow mechanisms are normal in NTG, aqueous suppressants simply decrease aqueous volume but that this is matched and corrected for by the pressure-dependent trabecular meshwork outflow, resulting in minimal net benefit with regard to IOP. Drugs that target the uveoscleral pathway may be ideal for NTG.

Prostaglandin analogs do not appear to change the blood velocity in retrobulbar vessels.[56] Alpha-2-agonists also do not appear to affect blood flow to the optic nerve making them potentially useful in NTG. Carbonic anhydrase inhibitors, although less effective in lowering IOP than other drugs, may potentially increase ocular blood flow by their effect on carbon dioxide induced vasodilatation.[57]

Calcium channel blockers

Calcium channel blockers are thought to decrease vasospasm and increase capillary dilatation thereby facilitating blood supply to the ONH. Despite some encouraging evidence in the literature,[58,59] the benefits of oral nifedipine (and other calcium channel blockers) on the clinical course of NTG is unclear and a continued matter for speculation.

One study reported no apparent difference in the stability of the visual fields or optic disc appearance for NTG patients on calcium channel blockers (for non-ophthalmic conditions) compared with those on no such drugs.[60] In contrast, another study reported that fewer NTG patients on calcium channel blocker therapy had less evidence of glaucoma progression than NTG patients not taking calcium channel blockers.[61]

Without definitive evidence it is difficult to make hard-and-fast recommendations regarding the use of these powerful drugs purely for their effect on glaucoma. There are significant side effects of therapy, in particular systemic hypotension. Many patients complain of troublesome foot swelling with even small doses of these drugs. Patients with documented progression despite optimal IOPs may benefit from treatment with calcium channel blockers, but only after appropriate and frank discussion with the patient.

Differential diagnosis

Intermittently high IOPs can result in significant glaucoma despite a normal IOP on formal assessment in the clinic. Intermittent angle-closure glaucoma, uveitic glaucoma or 'burnt-out' pigmentary glaucoma can all cause prolonged but self-limiting raised IOP. Such conditions can usually be detected by eliciting a careful history, thorough slit lamp examination and gonioscopy.

Non-glaucomatous conditions that mimic normal-tension glaucoma

Any condition that gives an optic nerve appearance consistent with glaucoma or a visual-field abnormality with a normal IOP can be confused with NTG.

Physiological optic disc cupping is a diagnosis of exclusion once a search for glaucoma has been thoroughly exhausted.

Several congenital anomalies such as ONH colobomas, nerve head drusen, optic disc pits and tilted or oblique discs may produce visual-field defects that can be confused with NTG.

Anterior ischemic optic neuropathy (AION) can result in a disc with a cup. There are two types of AION: the arteritic form caused by giant cell arteritis (GCA), and a non-arteritic form associated with microvasculopathies, such as hypertension, diabetes and arteriosclerosis. AION generally involves patients older than 50 years. It classically presents as a sudden, painless loss of vision in one eye in conjunction with optic disc swelling. Visual-field loss is often localized to one hemifield leaving an altitudinal field defect. After the initial disc swelling, pallor usually ensues after 4–6 weeks. In some cases of resolved arteritic AION the optic disc can be left with an appearance consistent with glaucomatous cupping. The classical patient with GCA is elderly with symptoms of headache, scalp tenderness and jaw claudication with an elevated ESR or C-reactive protein. Cupping is generally not a feature of non-arteritic AION[62] but it can be seen in the aftermath of the arteritic variant.[63]

Any cause of ischemia to the ONH may infrequently result in cupping. Retinal embolic disease could be mistaken for NTG. Symptoms are usually acute loss of vision or visual field and evidence of emboli or attenuated retinal vessels. The blood supply to the ONH may also be compromised in the presence of severe transient blood loss (e.g. after trauma) or blood dyscrasias (e.g. sickle cell disease).

When to scan patients; neurological conditions that mimic normal-tension glaucoma

The clinician should always be on the look out for compressive lesions resulting in a field defect with optic nerve changes consistent with NTG. Neurological conditions that could be confused with NTG include meningiomas, pituitary adenomas, craniopharyngiomas and Leber's optic neuropathy.

One case series[64] demonstrated lesions compressing the anterior visual pathway in 16 patients with 'normal' IOP. The pattern of field loss in most of their patients was a bitemporal defect with loss of Snellen acuity out of proportion to the extent of the optic cupping.

Another study documented data on 52 eyes of 29 patients with NTG and 44 eyes of 28 control patients with compressive lesions.[65] They found that none of the patients diagnosed with glaucoma had evidence of a mass lesion on imaging. Patients with compressive disease tended to be younger, had worse visual acuities, had visual fields that respected the vertical midline and displayed neuroretinal rim pallor.

Detailed assessments of the optic disc, visual acuity, visual fields and the age of the patient should provide ample information to rule out compressive lesion of the optic nerves or chiasm and NTG.

If everything fits and the patient conforms absolutely into a classical description of NTG then imaging is not required. The visual acuity should be normal. The remaining NRR should be of a normal healthy color. If it is pale then scan the patient.

The degree of optic disc cupping should correspond to the amount of visual-field loss. A discrepancy should prompt imaging. Scrutinize the visual field and determine whether the defect obeys the vertical midline. If there is any doubt then neuroimaging is prudent.

In general it is wise to scan a patient who is under 50 years of age, if their optic disc is swollen or pale, if the visual field obeys the vertical midline or if the visual acuity is reduced.

References

1. Von Graefe A. Amaursos mit Sehnervenexcavation. Archiv Ophthalmol 1857; 68: 389.
2. Lee BL, Renuka B, Weinreb RN. The definition of normal-tension glaucoma. J Glaucoma 1998; 7: 366–371.
3. Caprioli J. Editorial: the treatment of normal-tension glaucoma. Am J Ophthalmol 1998; 126: 578–581.
4. Sommer A. Glaucoma: facts and fancies. Eye 1996; 10: 295–301.
5. Klein BEK, Klein R, Sponsel WE, *et al.* Prevalence of glaucoma: the Beaver Dam Eye Study. Ophthalmology 1992; 99: 1499–504.
6. Sommer A, Tielsch JM, Katz J, *et al.* Relationship between intraocular pressure and primary open angle glaucoma among white and black Americans. The Baltimore Eye Survey. Arch Ophthalmol 1991; 109: 1090–1095.
7. Klein BEK, Klein R, Sponsel WE, *et al.* Prevalence of glaucoma: the Beaver Dam Eye Study. Ophthalmology 1992; 99: 1499–504.
9. Levene R. Low tension glaucoma: a critical review and new material. Surv Ophthalmol 1980; 61: 621–664.
8. Orgul S, Gaspar AZ, Hendrickson P, Flammer J. Comparison of the severity of normal-tension glaucoma in men and women. Ophthalmologica 1994; 208: 142–144.
10. Kaiser HJ, Schoetzau A, Stumpfig D, Flammer J. Blood-flow velocities of the extraocular vessels in patients with high-tension and normal-tension primary open-angle glaucoma. Am J Ophthalmol 1997; 123: 320–327.
11. Nicolela MT, Hnik P, Drance SM. Scanning laser Doppler flowmeter study of retinal and optic disk blood flow in glaucomatous patients. Am J Ophthalmol 1996; 122: 775–783.
12. Yamazaki Y, Drance SM. The relationship between progression of visual-field defects and retrobulbar circulation in patients with glaucoma. Am J Ophthalmol 1997; 123: 287–295.
13. Cellini M, Possati GL, Sbrocca M, Caramazza N. Correlation between visual field and color Doppler parameters in chronic open angle glaucoma. Int Ophthalmol 1996; 20: 215–219.
14. Harris A, Joos K, Kay M, *et al.* Acute IOP elevation with scleral suction: effects on retrobulbar hemodyamics. Br J Ophthalmol 1996; 80: 1055–1059.
15. Harris A, Spaeth G, Wilson R, *et al.* Nocturnal ophthalmic arterial hemodyamics in primary open-angle glaucoma. J Glaucoma 1997; 6: 170–174.
16. Emre M, Orgul S, Gugleta K, Flammer J. Ocular blood flow alteration in glaucoma is related to systemic vascular dysregulation. Br J Ophthalmol 2004; 88: 662–666.
17. Broadway DC, Drance SM. Glaucoma and vasospasm. Br J Ophthalmol 1998; 82: 862–870.
18. Gasser P. Ocular vasospasm: a risk factor in the pathogenesis of low-tension glaucoma. Int Ophthalmol 1989; 13: 281–290.
19. Hayreh SS, Zimmerman MB, Podhajsky P, Alward WL. Nocturnal arterial hypotension and its role in optic nerve head and ocular ischemic disorders. Am J Ophthalmol 1994; 15(117): 603–624.
20. Muzyka M, Nizankowska MH, Koziorowska M, Zajac-Pytrus H. Occurrence of nocturnal arterial hypotension in patients with primary open-angle glaucoma and normal tension glaucoma. Klln Oczna 1997; 99: 109 113.

21. Kaiser HJ, Flammer J, Graf T, Stumpfig D. Systemic blood pressure in glaucoma patients. Graefes Arch Clin Exp Ophthalmol 1993; 231: 677–680.
22. Plange N, Kaup M, Daneljan L, Predel HG, Remky A, Arend O. 24-h blood pressure monitoring in normal tension glaucoma: night-time blood pressure variability. J Hum Hypertens 2006; 20: 137–142.
23. Meyer JH, Brandi-Dohrn J, Funk J. Twenty-four hour blood pressure monitoring in normal tension glaucoma. Br J Ophthalmol 1996; 80: 864–867.
24. Graham SL, Drance SM, Wijsman K, *et al.* Ambulatory blood pressure monitoring in glaucoma. The nocturnal dip. Ophthalmology 1995; 102: 61–69.
25. Choi J, Jeong J, Cho HS, Kook MS. Effect of nocturnal blood pressure reduction on circadian fluctuation of mean ocular perfusion pressure: a risk factor for normal tension glaucoma. Invest Ophthalmol Vis Sci 2006; 47: 831–836.
26. Morad Y, Sharon E, Hefetz L, Nemet P. Corneal thickness and curvature in normal tension glaucoma. Am J Ophthalmol 1998; 125: 164–168.
27. Copt RP, Thomas R, Mermoud A. Corneal thickness in ocular hypertension, primary open-angle glaucoma, and normal tension glaucoma. Arch Ophthalmol 1999; 117: 14–16.
28. Ehlers N, Bramsen T, Sperling S. Applanation tonometry and central corneal thickness. Acta Ophthalmol (Copenh) 1975; 53: 34–43.
29. Whitacre MM, Stein RA, Hassanein K. The effect of corneal thickness on applanation tonometry. Am J Ophthalmol 1993; 15: 592–596.
30. Cartwright MJ, Anderson DR. Correlation of asymmetric damage with asymmetric intraocular pressure in normal-tension glaucoma (low-tension glaucoma). Arch Ophthalmol 1988; 106: 898–900.
31. Orgul S, Flammer J. Interocular visual field and intraocular pressure asymmetries in normal tension glaucoma. Eur J Ophthalmol 1994; 4: 199–201.
32. Crichton A, Drance SM, Douglas GR, Schulzer M. Unequal intraocular pressure and its relation to asymmetric visual-field defects in low tension glaucoma. Ophthalmology 1989; 96: 1312–1314.
33. Choi J, Kim KH, Jeong J, Cho HS, Lee CH, Kook MS. Circadian fluctuation of mean ocular perfusion pressure is a consistent risk factor for normal-tension glaucoma. Invest Ophthalmol Vis Sci 2007; 48: 104–111.
34. Nakagami T, Yamazaki Y, Hayamizu F. Prognostic factors for progression of visual field damage in patients with normal-tension glaucoma. Jpn J Ophthalmol 2006; 50: 38–43.
35. Bhandari A, Crabb DP, Poinoosawmy D, *et al.* Effect of surgery on visual field progression in normal tension glaucoma. Ophthalmology 1997; 104: 1131–1137.
36. Collaborative Normal-Tension Glaucoma Study Group. Comparison of glaucomatous progression between untreated patients with normal-tension glaucoma and patients with therapeutically reduced intraocular pressures. Am J Ophthalmol 1998; 126: 487–497.
36. Caprioli J, Spaeth GL. Comparison of the optic nerve head in high- and low-tension glaucoma. Arch Ophthalmol 1985; 103: 1145–1149.
37. Tuulonen A, Airaksinen PJ. Optic disc size in exfoliative, primary open angle, and low-tension glaucoma. Arch Ophthalmol 1992; 10: 211–213.
38. Jonas JB. Size of glaucomatous discs. Ger J Ophthalmol 1992; 1: 41–44.
39. Javitt JC, Spaeth GL, Katz LJ, *et al.* Acquired pits of the optic nerve. Increased prevalence in patients with low-tension glaucoma. Ophthalmology 1990; 97: 1038–1043.
40. Aduaguba C, Ugurlu S, Caprioli J. Acquired pits of the optic nerve in glaucoma: prevalence and associated visual field loss. Acta Ophthalmol Scand 1998; 76: 272–277.
41. Chumbley LC, Brubaker RF. Low-tension glaucoma. Am J Ophthalmol 1976; 81: 76.
42. Tuulonen A, Airaksinene PF, Alanko HI. Optic disc size in eyes with and without an optic disc hemorrhage. Invest Ophthalmol Vis Sci 1992; 33(suppl): 883.
43. Kitazawa Y, Shirato S, Yamamoto T. Optic disc hemorrhage in low-tension glaucoma. Ophthalmology 1986; 93: 853–857.

44. Gloster J. Incidence of optic disc haemorrhages in chronic simple glaucoma and ocular hypertension. Br J Ophthalmol 1981; 65: 452–456.
45. Airaksinen PJ, Mustonen E, Alanko HI. Optic disc hemorrhages. Analysis of stereophotographs and clinical data of 112 patients. Arch Ophthalmol 1981; 99: 1795–1801.
46. Sugiyama K, Tomita G, Kitazawa Y, et al. The association of optic disc hemorrhage with retinal nerve fiber layer defect and peripapillary atrophy in normal-tension glaucoma. Ophthalmology 1997; 104: 1926–1933.
47. Drance SM. Disc hemorrhages in the glaucomas. Surv Ophthalmol 1989; 33: 331–337.
48. Jonas JB, Bennis S. Localised wedge shaped defects of the retinal nerve fibre layer in glaucoma. Br J Ophthalmol 1994; 78: 285–290.
49. Yamazaki Y, Koide C, Miyazawa T, et al. Comparison of retinal nerve-fiber layer in high- and normal-tension glaucoma. Graefes Arch Clin Exp Ophthalmol 1991; 229: 517–520.
50. Uchida H, Ugurlu S, Caprioli J. Increasing peripapillary atrophy is associated with progressive glaucoma. Ophthalmology 1998; 105: 1541–1545.
51. Drance SM, Douglas GR, Airaksinen PJ, et al. Diffuse visual field loss in chronic open-angle and low-tension glaucoma. Am J Ophthalmol 1987; 104: 577–580.
52. Samuelson TW, Spaeth GL. Focal and diffuse visual field defects: their relationship to intraocular pressure. Ophthalmic Surg 1993; 24: 519–525.
53. Hitchings RA, Anderton SA. A comparative study of visual field defects seen in patients with low-tension glaucoma and chronic simple glaucoma. Br J Ophthalmol 1983; 67: 818–821.
54. Caprioli J, Spaeth GL. Comparison of visual field defects in the low-tension glaucomas with those in the high-tension glaucomas. Am J Ophthalmol 1984; 97: 730–737.
55. Koseki N, Araie M, Suzuki Y, Yamagami J. Visual field damage proximal to fixation in normal- and high-tension glaucoma eyes. Jpn J Ophthalmol 1995; 39: 274–283.
56. Nicolela MT, Buckley AR, Walman BE, Drance SM. A comparative study of the effects of timolol and latanoprost on blood flow velocity of the retrobulbar vessels. Am J Ophthalmol 1996; 122: 784–789.
57. Harris A, Joos K, Kay M, et al. Acute IOP elevation with scleral suction: effects on retrobulbar hemodyamics. Br J Ophthalmol 1996; 80: 1055–1059.
58. Hirooka K, Baba T, Fujimura T, Shiraga F. Prevention of visual-field defect progression with angiotensin-converting enzyme inhibitor in eyes with normal-tension glaucoma. Am J Ophthalmol 2006; 142: 523–525.
59. Gasser P. Ocular vasospasm: a risk factor in the pathogenesis of low-tension glaucoma. Int Ophthalmol 1989; 13: 281–290.
60. Liu S, Araujo SV, Spaeth GL, et al. Lack of effect of calcium channel blockers on open-angle glaucoma. J Glaucoma 1996; 5: 187–190.
61. Netland PA, Chaturvedi N, Dryer EB. Calcium channel blockers in the management of low-tension and open-angle glaucoma. Am J Ophthalmol 1993; 15: 608–613.
62. Hayreh SS, Jonas JB. Optic disc morphology after arteritic anterior ischemic optic neuropathy. Ophthalmology 2001; 108: 1586–1594.
63. Jonas JB, Xu L. Optic disc morphology in eyes after nonarteritic anterior ischemic optic neuropathy. Invest Ophthalmol Vis Sci 1993; 34: 2260–2265.
64. Kupersmith MJ, Krohn D. Cupping of the optic disc with compressive lesions of the anterior visual pathway. Ann Ophthalmol 1984; 16: 948–953.
65. Greenfield DS, Siatkowski RM, Glaser JS, et al. The cupped disc. Who needs neuroimaging? Ophthalmology 1998; 105: 1866–1874.

Chapter 21

Secondary open-angle glaucoma

The diagnosis of POAG is a diagnosis of exclusion. A variety of ocular, systemic, and congenital disorders can result in an elevated IOP and the clinician must make a conscious effort to detect the presence of any causative local or more widespread pathology.

Identification of a secondary glaucoma will have an impact on treatment, management options and prognosis. Thorough history and examination are key to diagnosing a secondary glaucoma. The best technique to use is to consciously ask oneself whether there is any evidence of the conditions listed within this chapter. Documenting these negatives may be beneficial.

Pseudoexfoliation syndrome

Pseudoexfoliation (PXF) syndrome occurs due to diffuse deposition of white dandruff-like material within the anterior segment of the eye. The PXF material results from abnormal protein synthesis and has been recovered from the corneal endothelium, the lens capsule, the ciliary zonules and the trabecular meshwork (TM). The PXF material clogs up the TM and causes impaired aqueous outflow with raised IOP. Pseudoexfoliation glaucoma is the term applied to glaucoma associated with the raised IOP secondary to PXF syndrome.

PXF occurs throughout the world but it is particularly prevalent in Scandinavian races.[1,2] Although the syndrome is more prevalent in women, pseudoexfoliative glaucoma tends to occur in both sexes equally.[3]

The prevalence of PXF syndrome increases significantly with age, first appearing after the fifth decade and reaching a maximum incidence in the seventh decade of life. Approximately one half of the cases of PXF syndrome are unilateral or asymmetric between the two eyes.[4–6] Most cases become bilateral eventually, usually within 10 years of detection. Heredity does not seem to be a factor in the development of PXF syndrome, and no underlying systemic predilection to the disorder has been found.

The incidence of PXF syndrome in the open-angle glaucoma population varies from 3% in most populations to 75% in Sweden.[7] Patients with PXF syndrome have a greater risk of developing glaucomatous damage.[8] Among patients with PXF, 5% develop elevated IOP within 5 years of diagnosis, increasing to 15% of patients within 10 years.[9] In one study, 16% of PXF patients required treatment upon presentation while 44% received therapy over the next 15 years.[10] In most cases, IOP elevation develops in the fellow eye within 6 years.[11]

Glaucoma occurs in approximately 7–20% of patients with PXF syndrome, and the IOP in PXF patients tends to be higher and more difficult to control than in patients with POAG.[8] Such patients may also have significant IOP fluctuations.[12]

Arguably, PXF ocular hypertension does not exist. Patients with raised IOP and PXF will almost certainly go on to develop glaucoma which may progress rapidly. They should be treated as glaucoma cases and appropriate IOP lowering initiated.

Hypoperfusion of the iris vessels is apparent on iris fluorescein angiography, and neovascular-like clumps of iris vessels are sometimes observed.[13,14] The role that these findings play in PXF syndrome remains unclear.

Clinical findings

PXF material is usually found on most of the structures of the anterior segment of the eye, including the corneal endothelium, the pupillary border (Fig. 5.4), and the anterior surface of the iris. Transillumination defects of the iris are present, beginning at the pupillary border and extending to the midperipheral iris. The pupillary border of the iris may take on a moth-eaten appearance on retroillumination.

The distinctive appearance of gray–white granular material on the anterior lens capsule is the hallmark of this disorder. A central translucent zone is often surrounded by a clear zone that corresponds to an area of rubbing on the anterior lens capsule by the posterior surface of the iris at the pupillary border (Fig. 5.8).

Pigment dispersion into the AC may occur after pharmacological mydriasis, and a post-dilation pressure spike is common.[14,15] Pigment in the TM may represent the earliest sign of PXF syndrome, and its appearance may predate the capsular lens changes.[14] Sampaolesi's line, a pigmented line anterior to Schwalbe's line, can often be seen in PXF syndrome.

PXF patients have weaker ciliary zonules which may make cataract surgery more technically challenging with an increased risk of complication.

Treatment and management

IOP is often higher in PXF glaucoma and is more refractory to treatment compared to POAG. Medical treatment with the full spectrum of topical ocular hypotensives should be initiated.

Argon laser trabeculoplasty (ALT) has been shown to be very effective in lowering IOP in PXF glaucoma.[16,17] Apraclonidine (Iopidine) can be administered prophylactically to prevent post-laser IOP spikes.[18] Filtration surgery can also be performed in the treatment of PXF glaucoma and demonstrates results similar to those reported for patients with POAG.

Pigmentary glaucoma

Pigmentary dispersion syndrome (PDS) is characterized by the liberation of pigment particles from the posterior iris pigment epithelium.[19] The pigment particles are carried by aqueous convection currents and deposited on the corneal endothelium, anterior surface of the iris, anterior surface of the crystalline lens, ciliary zonules and the TM. Elevated IOP can result from the obstruction of aqueous outflow by pigment granules that clog the TM.[20] Elevated IOP can lead to glaucomatous damage to the optic nerve (pigmentary glaucoma).

Most patients with pigmentary dispersion are white, and the disorder is rare in black or Asian people. PDS typically affects young myopes who are anatomically predisposed by having a posterior concave iris contour. Men and women have similar rates of PDS, however, pigmentary glaucoma is more common in males. The age of onset is slightly younger in men, 35–45 years compared to a decade later for women, especially in higher degrees of myopia.[19-22] Pigmentary glaucoma accounts for 1.0–1.5% of all glaucomas.[19] The liberation of this pigment appears to diminish with time and thus the incidence of pigmentary glaucoma decreases with advancing age.

One study[23] found that the risk of developing pigmentary glaucoma from pigment dispersion syndrome was 10% at 5 years and 15% at 15 years. Young, myopic men were most likely to have pigmentary glaucoma and an IOP greater than 21 mmHg at initial examination was associated with an increased risk of conversion.

Clinicopathology

PDS is characterized by a loss of pigment from the pigment epithelium of the iris. The loss of pigment manifests as iris transillumination defects in the midperipheral to peripheral zone of the iris (Fig. 5.7). The AC angle in pigment dispersion is deeper and appears to bow posteriorly in a concave configuration. This posterior curve of the iris theoretically results in mechanical contact of the posterior iris surface with the ciliary zonules every time the pupil reacts.[24,25]

The mechanism of the raised IOP in PDS is not completely understood. Pigment granules accumulate in the trabecular meshwork and eventually cause a dysfunction of trabecular endothelial cells.[26,27] These cells are responsible for the phagocytosis of pigment granules and cellular debris. With the build-up of pigment and cellular debris, aqueous outflow becomes obstructed. Patients with pigmentary glaucoma may release large batches of iris pigment when changes occur in pupil size or on exercise. This acute release of pigment can cause dramatic elevations in the IOP. Dense pigmentation of the TM may occur in the absence of elevated IOP and is not always indicative of pathology.

Iris fluorescein angiography studies in pigmentary dispersion have demonstrated vascular hypoperfusion of the iris, decreased iris vessels and leakage of fluorescein, especially at the pupillary border.

Clinical findings

The classical sign of PDS is the presence of pigment on the corneal endothelium called a Krukenberg spindle (Fig. 5.1). Small specks of pigment may be seen floating within the aqueous convection currents of the AC. Spoke-like radial transillumination defects are seen in the iris (Fig. 5.7). Gonioscopy reveals a wide open angle, sometimes a concave appearance to the iris and diffuse pigmentation of the TM. A pigmented Schwalbe's line can sometimes be observed (Sampaolesi's line) (Fig. 6.10).

The patient is usually asymptomatic, but may experience symptoms of blurred vision or halos if they suffer significant IOP spikes. Pharmacological mydriasis can cause an acute pressure rise and thus such patients should have their IOPs rechecked after dilating.

Patients with PDS and a normal IOP with no signs of glaucoma need regular IOP checks to detect IOP elevation. If they are going to get glaucoma it will be the high-pressure variety and should thus be picked up by regularly checking IOP. Potentially such follow-up may occur at their own optician.

Treatment and management

Medical therapy is the first line of treatment and the full spectrum of medication may be used.

Pilocarpine is quite effective in lowering the IOP in patients with pigmentary glaucoma both by the effect on the trabecular meshwork (and thus outflow) but also because it theoretically decreases iridozonular contact minimizing the continued pigment liberation. However this drug is poorly tolerated in younger patients and is thus of limited value.

Laser trabeculoplasty, either ALT or SLT, is a viable and highly efficacious option for patients with pigmentary glaucoma.

Laser peripheral iridotomy (LPI) has been advocated as a prophylactic measure in this condition. The theory is that the LPI relieves the reverse pupillary block which is responsible for the posterior bowing of the iris. By stopping this, the iris zonule contact is prevented and the pigment liberation stops. This treatment is controversial and is not uniformly used. It makes sense to use this if the iris is markedly concave in appearance. It must be remembered that the effect will be delayed as the eye will take time to clear the pigment already within the trabecular meshwork.

Uveitic glaucoma

Intraocular inflammation may result in both secondary open- and closed-angle glaucoma. Raised IOP is seen more commonly in cases with evidence of chronic inflammation rather than a one-off inflammatory episode.[28]

The etiology of uveitis is often never fully elucidated, but the condition can be associated with certain systemic diseases, such as sarcoidosis, systemic lupus erythematosus, ankylosing spondylitis, syphilis, tuberculosis, Reiter's syndrome and rheumatoid arthritis.[29,30] The herpes viridae are particular culprits for causing a uveitis which can lead to secondary glaucoma. Uveitis can occur after trauma or intraocular surgery, or may be due to a primary ocular disorder such as Fuchs' heterochromic iridocyclitis or glaucomatocyclitic crisis (Posner-Schlossman syndrome).

Mechanisms of elevated intraocular pressure in uveitis:

- Clogging of trabecular meshwork (TM) by inflammatory cells and debris
- Chronic scarring of outflow channels
- Chronic steroid use
- Inflammatory edema and dysfunction of the trabecular meshwork (trabeculitis)

- Peripheral anterior synechiae (PAS) formation causing angle closure
- Iris bombé from 360° posterior synechiae
- Angle neovascularization from retinal or iridial ischemic processes

Clinicopathology

Inflammation within the eye causes breakdown of the blood–aqueous barrier resulting in liberation of protein and inflammatory cells into the vitreous and aqueous. Inflammatory debris is swept into the drainage angle via normal aqueous flow and causes an obstruction at the TM with consequent raised IOP. Trabeculitis (inflammation of the TM) which is often associated with viral etiologies can block aqueous outflow and raise IOP.

This inflammatory blockage is initially reversible once the inflammation has settled, however with chronic or repeated episodes structural changes occur in the drainage mechanism causing permanent damage (such as TM scarring or PAS) and chronically elevated IOP.

Clinical findings

The uveitis may be active or quiescent at the time of assessment. Look for signs of previous inflammatory episodes such as iris atrophy, PAS, posterior synechiae, old keratic precipitates, cataract and pigment on the corneal endothelium.

Treatment and management

The inflammation has to be controlled as a first step to arrest the pathological process. Cycloplegics and topic anti-inflammatory agents (usually corticosteroids) are the mainstay of treatment. Cycloplegics aid comfort, break down any posterior synechiae and stabilize the iridial vasculature. Topical corticosteroids inhibit the inflammatory response and decrease capillary permeability, thus normalizing the blood–aqueous barrier and reducing the release of inflammatory cells and protein.

Aqueous suppressors, such as beta-blockers, alpha-agonists and topical carbonic anhydrase inhibitors, can be used to achieve IOP reduction. Miotic agents should be avoided because they can exacerbate inflammation and increase the likelihood of posterior synechiae formation. Peripheral iridotomy is indicated if a risk of pupillary block from 360° of posterior synechiae exists.

Prostaglandin use in uveitic glaucoma is controversial. The prostaglandin pathway is key to the genesis of inflammation and some clinicians believe that use of agonist agents may exacerbate inflammation or risk cystoid macular edema. Certainly prostaglandins should not be used as first-line therapy. If the IOP remains uncontrolled and there are no active signs of excessive inflammation then they may be introduced cautiously. If the inflammation worsens or macular thickness increases they should immediately discontinued.

Glaucomatocyclitic crisis

Glaucomatocyclitic crisis (Posner-Schlossman syndrome) is a condition whereby the patient suffers recurrent episodes of mild anterior uveitis associated with marked IOP elevation. Patients tend to be relatively asymptomatic despite a very high IOP.

The high IOP is most probably caused by a trabeculitis. The disorder is unfortunately recurrent in nature, and the patient should be monitored for the development of visual-field defects and optic nerve damage. The acute episode is treated with topical corticosteroids, beta-blockers, alpha-agonists and topical carbonic anhydrase inhibitors.

Topical prostaglandins, miotic agents and laser trabeculoplasty should be avoided.

Fuchs' heterochromic iridocyclitis

Fuchs' heterochromic iridocyclitis is a form of anterior uveitis which is associated with the development of secondary cataract and glaucoma. Most cases are unilateral, affect men and women equally, and have an onset in the fourth decade of life.[31] Raised IOP is seen in 13–59% of patients.[32] Clinically there is a mild anterior uveitis with only minimal cell activity and flare. The endothelium classically shows the presence of round or stellate keratitic precipitates scattered throughout the whole endothelial surface. The iris may be hypochromic and have gray–white nodules on its anterior surface.[32]

The exact etiology of the elevated IOP is poorly understood. The angles are usually open and synechiae do not form. It is probable that the chronic unremitting low-grade inflammatory process results in scarring of the TM. Treatment options include topical beta-blocking agents, alpha-agonists, carbonic anhydrase inhibitors, corticosteroids and cycloplegic agents to treat the uveitis component. Glaucoma surgery is often required in such cases.

Angle-recession glaucoma

Angle recession occurs when a blunt object impacts the front of the eye and causes a forceful posterior dislocation of the ocular contents. After the force is dissipated the cornea and sclera bounce rapidly back to their original shape but the greater density of the crystalline lens prevents it from returning as quickly. This causes an opposing force that can result in a tear between the longitudinal and circular muscles of the ciliary body.

The area of recession may be localized or it may be extensive involving the whole circumference of the angle. The actual recession itself does not cause the problem directly, although it does result in less opening tractional force on the trabecular meshwork. Instead it acts as a surrogate marker for concurrent damage to the TM which is actually what causes the glaucoma.

Gonioscopy reveals widening of the ciliary body band in one or more quadrants of the angle in the affected eye. In cases of 360° recession, detection is facilitated by comparison to the fellow eye. The greater the circumference and depth of the angle recess, the greater the likelihood that a secondary glaucoma will eventually develop.[33] In a 10-year prospective study of patients with angle recession an incidence of 9% for the development of glaucoma was found.[34]

Management

Medical management of traumatic or angle-recession glaucoma consists of aqueous-suppressing agents, such as topical beta-blockers, alpha-agonists and carbonic anhydrase inhibitors. Angle laser is usually inadvisable. In the acute trauma situation prostaglandins are contraindicated, but in the setting of late-onset glaucoma they may be tried. Filtering surgery may be required in medically uncontrollable cases.

Glaucoma associated with hyphema

Traumatic hyphema secondary to blunt ocular trauma may be associated with an acute rise in IOP secondary to blood obstructing the TM. The greater the amount of blood in the AC the greater the likelihood of IOP elevation. Re-bleeding, which often occurs 3–5 days after the original injury tends to be problematic as regards the risk of significant IOP elevation.

Management

Management of elevated IOP secondary to hyphema is by use of topical beta-blockers, alpha-agonists, oral or intravenous carbonic anhydrase inhibitors and oral or intravenous hyperosmotic agents. Strong cycloplegics, such as 1% atropine, may be used to prevent posterior synechiae and limit iris movement. Hospitalization of young children with strict bed rest does not seem to prevent the likelihood of a rebleed[35,36] but nonetheless it appears a prudent measure. Some studies have demonstrated that the use of oral aminocaproic acid administered 100 mg/kg every 4 hours, along with rest, decreased the possibility of a rebleed.[37] Patients should be followed on a daily basis and IOP monitored until the hyphema has fully resolved.[38] The original injury must have been significant and thus these patients are at risk of developing late raised IOP due to concurrent initially subclinical trabecular meshwork damage.

Surgical evacuation of the hyphema is sometimes necessary, but evidence suggests that a delay is advisable to minimize complications. Surgery is indicated in cases of intractable pain, severely elevated IOP (50–60 mmHg for 4–5 days), blood staining of the cornea and hyphemas that remain longer than 9 days.[39]

Glaucoma associated with intraocular hemorrhage

Vitreous hemorrhage may result in a ghost cell secondary glaucoma. Red blood cells gradually degenerate over a few weeks to form inflexible ghost cells. These ghost cells usually remain within the vitreous cavity but if the anterior hyaloid face has been breached they can migrate forward into the AC and block the TM. This process may occur months after the initial bleed. The ghost cells in the AC are visualized as tan color specks floating in the aqueous currents.

Management

Ghost cell glaucoma is initially treated medically. If IOP cannot be adequately controlled, surgical evacuation of the cells in the AC may be required or even vitrectomy to clear the source of the blood.

References

1. Dell WM. The epidemiology of the pseudoexfoliation syndrome. J Am Optom Assoc 1985; 56: 113–119.
2. Ohrt V, Nehen JH. The incidence of glaucoma capsulare based on a Danish hospital material. Acta Ophthalmol 1981; 59: 888–893.
3. Henry JC, Krupin T, Schmitt M, *et al.* Long-term follow-up of pseudoexfoliation and the development of elevated intraocular pressure. Ophthalmology 1987; 94: 545–552.
4. Hiller R, Sperduto RO, Krueger DE. Pseudoexfoliation, intraocular pressure, and senile lens changes in a population-based survey. Arch Ophthalmol 1982; 100: 1080–1082.
5. Hansen E, Sellevold OJ. Pseudoexfoliation of the lens capsule. Development of the exfoliation syndrome. Acta Ophthalmol 1969; 47: 161–173.
6. Kozart DM, Yanoff M. Intraocular pressure status in 100 consecutive patients with exfoliation syndrome. Ophthalmology 1982; 89: 214–218.
7. Layden WE, Shaffer RN. Exfoliation syndrome. Am J Ophthalmol 1974; 78: 835–841.
8. Kozart DM, Yanoff M. Intraocular pressure status in 100 consecutive patients with exfoliation syndrome. Ophthalmology 1982; 89: 214–218.
9. Slagsvold JE. The follow-up in patients with pseudoexfoliation of the lens capsule with and without glaucoma. 2. The development of glaucoma in persons with pseudoexfoliation. Acta Ophthalmol 1986; 64: 241–245.
10. Jeng SM, Karger RA, Hodge DO, Burke JP, Johnson DH, Good MS. The risk of glaucoma in pseudoexfoliation syndrome. J Glaucoma 2007; 16: 117–121.
11. Brooks AM, Gillies WE. The presentation and prognosis of glaucoma in pseudoexfoliation of the lens capsule. Ophthalmology 1988; 95: 271–276.
12. Altintas O, Yuksel N, Karabas VL, Qaglar Y. Diurnal intraocular pressure variation in pseudoexfoliation syndrome. Eur J Ophthalmol 2004; 14: 495–500.
13. Brooks AM, Gillies WE. The development of microneovascular changes in the iris in pseudoexfoliation of the lens capsule. Ophthalmology 1987; 94: 1090–1097.
14. Krause U, Hine J, Frisius H. Pseudoexfoliation of the lens capsule and liberation of iris pigment. Acta Ophthalmol 1978; 56: 329–334.
15. Roth M, Epstein D. Exfoliation syndrome. Am J Ophthalmol 1980; 89: 477–481.
16. Lieberman ME, Hoskins HD, Hetherington J. Laser trabeculoplasty and the glaucomas. Ophthalmology 1983; 90: 790–795.
17. Higginbotham EJ, Richardson TM. Response of exfoliation glaucoma to laser trabeculoplasty. Br J Ophthalmol 1986: 70: 837–839.
18. Tuulonen A, Airaksinen PJ. Laser trabeculoplasty in simple and capsular glaucoma. Acta Ophthalmol 1983; 61: 1009–1015.
19. Sugar HS, Babour FA. Pigmentary glaucoma: a rare clinical entity. Am J Ophthalmol 1949; 32: 90–92.
20. Scheie HG, Cameron JD. Idiopathic atrophy of the epithelial layers of the iris and ciliary body. Arch Ophthalmol 1958; 59: 216–228.
21. Bick MW. Pigmentary glaucoma in females. Arch Ophthalmol 1957; 58: 483–494.

22. Berger A, Ritch R, McDermott JA, *et al*. Pigmentary dispersion, refraction and glaucoma. Invest Ophthalmol Vis Sci 1987; 28: 114–119.
23. Siddiqui Y, Ten Hulzen RD, Cameron JD, Hodge DO, Johnson DH. What is the risk of developing pigmentary glaucoma from pigment dispersion syndrome? Am J Ophthalmol 2003 Jun; 135(6): 794–799.
24. Davidson JA, Brubaker RE, Ilstrup DM. Dimension of the anterior chamber in pigment dispersion syndrome. Arch Ophthalmol 1983; 101: 81–83.
25. Campbell DG. Pigment dispersion syndrome and glaucoma: a new theory. Arch Ophthalmol 1979; 97: 1667–1672.
26. Lichter PR. Pigmentary glaucoma: current concepts. Trans Am Acad Ophthalmol Otolaryngol 1974; 78: 309–313.
27. Richter CU, Richardson TM, Grant WM. Pigmentary dispersion syndrome and pigmentary glaucoma: a prospective study of the natural history. Arch Ophthalmol 1986; 104: 211–215.
28. Herbert HM, Viswanathan A, Jackson H, Lightman SL. Risk factors for elevated intraocular pressure in uveitis. J Glaucoma 2004; 13: 96–99.
29. Smith ME, Zimmerman LE. Contusive angle recession in phacolytic glaucoma. Arch Ophthalmol 1965; 65: 799–804.
30. Jabs DA, Johns CJ. Ocular involvement in chronic sarcoidosis. Am J Ophthalmol 1986; 102: 297–301.
31. Franceschetti A. Heterochromic cyclitis (Fuchs' syndrome). Am J Ophthalmol 1955; 39: 50–58.
32. Liesgang TJ. Clinical features and prognosis in Fuchs' uveitis syndrome. Arch Ophthalmol 1982; 100: 1622–1626.
33. D'Ombrain AW. Traumatic monocular chronic glaucoma. Trans Ophthalmol Soc Aust 1945; 5: 116–121.
34. Kaufman JH, Tolpin DW. Glaucoma after traumatic angle recession. A ten-year prospective study. Am J Ophthalmol 1974; 78: 648–654.
35. Kaufmann JH, Tolpin DW. Glaucoma after traumatic angle recession. Am J Ophthalmol 1974; 78: 648–654.
36. Rakusin W. Traumatic hyphema. Am J Ophthalmol 1972; 74: 284–292.
37. Read J. Traumatic hyphema: surgical vs. medical management. Ann Ophthalmol 1975; 7: 659–670.
38. Kitazawa Y. Management of traumatic hyphema with glaucoma. Int Ophthalmol Clin 1979; 21: 167–181.
39. Rhee DJ, Pyfer MF (Eds). The Wills Eye Manual, Lippincott Wilkins & Wilkins, Philadelphia, 1999.

Chapter 22

Primary angle closure

Classification

Primary angle closure (PAC) occurs when the trabecular meshwork (TM) is physically blocked thus preventing trabecular aqueous outflow. The condition may be categorized according to the presence or absence of pupillary block and whether it is a primary or secondary phenomenon.

Pupillary block occurs when there is resistance to aqueous flow from the posterior chamber (PC) to the anterior chamber (AC) through the pupil. This resistance usually occurs at the pupil margin where the iris drapes over the anterior lens surface. As a pressure differential develops the peripheral iris moves forward (iris bombé) until it blocks the drainage angle (Fig. 6.9).

It is important to differentiate acute angle closure (AAC) from acute angle-closure glaucoma (AACG). In the former the IOP acutely increases as a result of closure of the drainage angle but the patient has no features of glaucoma (yet!). AACG implies that the raised IOP has caused glaucomatous optic neuropathy (optic disc changes and visual-field loss).

PAC with pupillary block occurs because there is a predisposing anatomic arrangement, i.e. a narrow angle. Again it is further necessary to distinguish PAC from primary angle-closure glaucoma (PACG) which occurs when the PAC results in optic nerve compromise and glaucoma. PAC may be further subdivided into suspect (potentially occludable angle), subacute, acute and chronic forms.

AAC can also occur in the absence of pupillary block, usually as a manifestation of the plateau iris syndrome. In this condition the central anterior chamber depth is normal, the iris plane is flat, the ciliary body is anatomically anterior, no ciliary sulcus is present and the peripheral AC angle is extremely narrow. Gonioscopy is key to making this diagnosis and reveals a very flat peripheral iris contour (like a plateau) which suddenly and sharply dips backwards/posteriorly before inserting into the ciliary body. The edge of the plateau lies close to the corneal endothelium thus leaving a very narrow angle.

Secondary angle closure (SAC) and secondary acute angle-closure glaucoma (SACG) are always associated with some other disease process. Thorough slit lamp examination of both eyes is usually sufficient to tell the two disease entities apart.

Epidemiology of primary angle-closure glaucoma

PACG is relatively uncommon in the US and accounts for less than 10% of all diagnosed cases of glaucoma.[1,2] In other populations, however, ACG occurs more frequently and may even exceed the incidence of open-angle glaucoma (OAG). Examples of populations with high incidences of ACG include the Mongoloid peoples of East Asia,[3] Greenland and Alaskan Eskimos,[4,5] and Orientals.[6] The prevalence of ACG within a particular population also depends on a number of variables. Primary among these are race, family history, age, sex and refractive error.

Risk factors for PAC include older age, female gender, Chinese ethnicity, all of which are associated with anatomical risk factors of central and/or peripherally shallow ACs (usually associated with a thicker, anteriorly-positioned lens), and a shorter axial length of the globe.[7]

Clinical background

Most cases of PAC are related to pupillary block and occur in eyes with narrow angles. As previously mentioned, a small degree of physiological relative pupillary block is always present in phakic individuals as the iris rests against the anterior surface of the lens. This iris–lens contact increases resistance of aqueous flow from the PC through the pupil and leads to an increase in the pressure behind the iris. If this pressure differential is sufficient the peripheral iris moves/bows forward. This peripheral iris ballooning (called iris bombé) can occlude the TM, impeding aqueous drainage and raising IOP.

Slight iris bombé may occur occasionally in normal eyes but it is not clinically significant as the angles are wide open and slight anterior movement will have no impact on angle dynamics and aqueous outflow. Only certain eyes with anatomical predisposition have AC depths small enough and angles narrow enough to undergo PAC.

When the pupil is mid dilated there is maximal pupil block occurring and the risk of precipitating angle closure is greatest. Such a situation may occur in environments where there is dim illumination. It may also be induced pharmacologically by a variety of systemic and topical medications. When the pupil is fully dilated, little contact occurs between the lens and the iris, and therefore minimum pupillary block is present.

When mydriatic drops are used the pupil dilates rapidly and goes through this high-risk mid-dilatation state rapidly with little risk of inducing PAC. However, as the dilating drops wear off the pupil slowly returns to its original state. The iris remains in the mid-dilated position for a longer period of time and the risk of inducing PAC is increased. With pharmacological dilatation using short-acting drugs (such as tropicamide) this typically occurs a few hours after the agent has been administered. If a patient is dilated and you are concerned that they have narrow angles it is prudent to check their IOP 2 hours after dilatation or make sure they know to reattend should their vision go blurry or they begin experiencing pain in the eye.

Acute primary angle closure

An acute angle closure attack is a true ophthalmic emergency, and requires immediate treatment in the hospital setting to prevent visual loss. Patients should be immediately and urgently referred to the hospital eye service for definitive management.

APAC is usually unilateral and occurs mostly in elderly hyperopic individuals.[8,9] Typical symptoms are the rapid onset of a red eye, pain, blurred vision, halos around lights, tearing, photophobia, nausea and vomiting.

Examination classically reveals ciliary injection, a shallow AC, a mid-dilated unreactive pupil, corneal edema and an IOP usually above 50 mmHg. Gonioscopy and slit lamp evaluation of the other eye often provide vital clues to whether the AAC is primary or secondary.

Conditions in the differential diagnosis include:

- POAG with unusually high IOP
- Glaucomatocyclitic crisis
- Neovascular glaucoma
- Plateau iris syndrome
- Malignant glaucoma
- Pigmentary dispersion syndrome/glaucoma
- Anterior chamber angle tumor or mass
- Uveitic glaucoma with or without secondary angle closure
- Phacomorphic glaucoma with secondary angle closure
- Iridocorneal endothelial syndrome

It is important that the above conditions are excluded as the pathogenesis of the IOP rise is very different and thus requires very different management.

Treatment of acute primary angle closure

Naturally acute management focuses upon reducing the IOP to prevent damage to the optic nerve. This involves the use of topical and systemic ocular hypotensive agents but an attempt must also be made to reverse the underlying problem, i.e. the pupil block.

Once the acute event is over prophylactic treatment should be carried out to prevent a further occurence. In addition treatment should be considered for the other eye as it will inevitably have a similar anatomic predisposition to angle closure.

Topical agents used are miotics (pilocarpine), beta-blockers, alpha-agonists, topical carbonic anhydrase inhibitors and steroids (to reduce inflammation). Intravenous CAI (e.g. acetazolamide) is usually given in the acute phase as nausea usually prohibits oral administration. The use of prostaglandin analogs in the presence of inflammation is controversial. If the IOP is non-responsive to other measures and the need for pressure reduction is urgent the risk–benefit profile for the use of one prostaglandin analog is in favor of their use.

Pilocarpine

Pilocarpine constricts the pupil, pulling the peripheral iris away from the trabecular meshwork and thus hopefully opening up the angle. When the IOP is higher than 40 mmHg, the pupillary sphincter muscle is often ischemic and unresponsive to topical miotic agents.[10,11] If pilocarpine is poured on to an eye with an extremely high IOP there may be no pharmacological benefit but a significant risk of systemic toxicity. Systemic toxicity manifests as a cholinergic crisis with nausea, vomiting, diarrhea, sweating, bradycardia and hypotension. Elderly patients are at particular risk.

Once the IOP has been reduced, normal blood flow returns to the iris sphincter, and it becomes responsive to pilocarpine therapy.[11] It makes sense to give a small dose of pilocarpine in the acute stage so that when the pupil sphincter becomes perfused once more there is a sufficient concentration of pilocarpine present to stimulate immediate miosis.[12–14]

Intravenous hyperosmotics such as mannitol should be used with caution especially in the elderly because of their systemic complications (dehydration, cardiovascular stress, disorientation, confusion, diarrhea and seizures).

An attack of AAC should not be considered broken until the IOP has returned to normal levels and the pupil is miotic. Gonioscopy should be carried out to ensure that the angle is now open. It also allows detection of peripheral anterior synechiae (PAS), which may have formed from appositional contact of the iris and TM. If the angle is not open, the IOP can rise again and the patient should be followed closely.

The patient should be maintained on 1 or 2% pilocarpine four times daily to both eyes until a laser peripheral iriditomy (LPI) is performed.

Laser peripheral iridotomy

An LPI should be performed within a few days once the eye is quiet and the pressure is stable. The cornea will also have cleared by that stage to a sufficient degree to allow adequate visualization of the iris and adequate laser treatment. An LPI should also be performed for the fellow eye as there is a likely anatomical predeliction in the unaffected eye. Naturally this decision should be based upon the gonioscopic findings of the other eye. For example, if the other eye is pseudophakic an LPI may not be required.

LPI is the definitive treatment for pupil block as it creates a connection between the anterior and posterior chambers thereby preventing any pressure differential and stopping anterior movement of the peripheral iris. Prophylactic LPI is indicated in all fellow eyes after an AAC attack in the opposite eye.[15] Intermittent and chronic angle-closure glaucoma are also considered to be indications for LPI.

Prognosis and follow-up

PAC patients should not be considered cured even after a successful LPI has been performed. These patients should be considered glaucoma suspects for life and receive appropriate follow-up care. The angle deepens immediately and stabilizes within the first 2 weeks after the laser.[16] No further change is seen over at least the first year. Along with IOP measurement and evaluating the iridotomy for patency, gonioscopy, visual fields and optic nerves should be monitored over the long term.

It is sometimes hard for the patency of the LPI to be fully confirmed. Although there may be an obvious transillumination defect (Fig. 22.1) it is not always easy to say for sure whether the hole has gone all the way through the iris or whether there is a thin residual membrane precluding flow. The clinician carrying out the laser treatment should document whether there was a pigment gush at the time of laser application. This pigment is liberated from the posterior layer of the iris and usually indicates a full-thickness puncture. Gonioscopy should be done before and after laser treatment to document whether the angle deepened.

Late-stage IOP rise may be a result of TM damage that occurred during the period of appositional closure. The development of OAG is also more common in these patients and so they warrant long-term follow-up to detect the onset of an OAG.

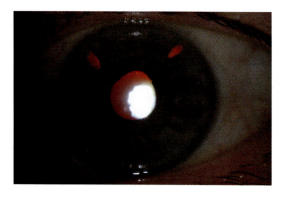

Figure 22.1 Color photograph clearly showing transillumination defects through patent peripheral iridotomies on retro-illumination.

Plateau iris syndrome

In this condition the central AC depth is normal, the iris plane is flat, the ciliary body is anatomically anterior, no ciliary sulcus is present and the peripheral anterior chamber angle is extremely narrow. Gonioscopy is key to making this diagnosis and reveals a very flat peripheral iris contour (like a plateau) which suddenly and sharply dips backwards before inserting into the ciliary body. The edge of the plateau lies close to the corneal endothelium thus leaving a very narrow angle. Pupillary dilation causes the peripheral iris to bunch up and occlude the small gap between the iris and the posterior cornea, closing the angle.

It is often impossible to be certain of the diagnosis based purely on gonioscopy. The diagnosis is only really confirmed when AAC occurs in the presence of a patent LPI. In this case pupil block has been eliminated as a causative factor leaving the plateau configuration as the likely cause.

Patients with plateau iris configuration typically have no symptoms until they develop an acute or subacute attack of PAC usually as a result of pharmacological or physiological pupillary dilatation. Their family members are also at risk of the condition.[17]

Treatment may be by the use of chronic miotic agents although this is less than ideal. Argon laser peripheral iridoplasty is highly effective in changing the contour of the peripheral iris and hopefully preventing AAC.[18] If the patient has a concurrent cataract then they should be considered for cataract extraction as this will change the angle anatomy and hopefully prevent any risk of PAC.

Argon laser peripheral iridoplasty

Argon laser burns applied to the peripheral iris can contract resulting in a change in peripheral iris contour. This technique can be used to open sections of the angle and may be effective as a treatment in cases of AAC secondary to plateau iris syndrome. It has also been used in the acute and chronic treatment of AAC with some success.[19]

Subacute angle closure

Patients undergo intermittent episodes of AAC. The angle becomes occluded and the IOP goes up transiently. The pupil block is spontaneously overcome, usually by movement of the iris (before it gets too ischemic) allowing the peripheral iris to fall back again and open the angle. That attack resolves spontaneously and the IOP goes back down to normal. It is just a matter of time before the AAC does not reverse itself and the IOP goes high enough to trigger the cascade into formal AAC. Sometimes repeated episodes of angle occlusion can result in stepwise PAS formation and eventual chronic angle closure (CAC).

Symptoms vary widely based on the level of IOP, the patient's pain threshold and level of awareness. Clinical signs of prior AAC attacks include PAS, glaucomflecken (small cyst-like areas in the anterior lens) and posterior synechiae in eyes with a narrow anterior chamber angle. A history of transient evening ocular pain, blurring of vision and halos may be elicited.

Chronic angle-closure glaucoma

Chronic primary ACG occurs secondary to permanent closure of a significant portion of the anterior chamber angle by PAS in an already narrow angle. Usually about 180–270° of the angle has to be occluded by PAS before aqueous outflow is impeded enough to raise IOP. Closure of the angle with PAS may progress slowly, a process which may be described as 'zipping' up of the angle.

The occludable angle

Prophylactic LPI is indicated in fellow eyes after a PAC attack in the opposite eye. Evidence of subacute angle closure attacks or chronic angle closure (the onset of PAS usually initially seen in the superior angle) are also considered indications for LPI.

When we know that the patient has had an IOP rise because of an AAC attack or if there are clear signs of previous attacks, the decision to proceed to LPI is clear.

The dilemma occurs when the gonioscopic appearance looks like the angle could close off but there is no evidence that this has occurred. LPI is not a completely innocuous intervention. Significant complications can occur, some of which may be sight threatening.

LPI is not indicated if the angle is not susceptible to spontaneous closure. The difficulty lies in deciding definitively which eyes are susceptible to this spontaneous closure. If there is no angle visible at all and the peripheral iris is almost in contact with the corneal endothelium then the decision becomes easier. There is a significant spectrum of angle appearance from definitely occludable (or even occluded), through possibly occludable to open. Even in the most experienced hands this distinction may be difficult.

As a general rule if there is less than 90° of the posterior (usually pigmented) trabecular meshwork visible, then the angle may be deemed occludable and a significant risk of potential future angle closure exists.[20]

Provocative testing has been used to try to trigger an AAC attack (or at least cause a detectable rise in IOP) in the hope of identifying eyes at risk for developing angle closure. These provocative tests have included the use of various pharmacological agents to dilate the pupil and other physiological tests, such as the dark room prone test.[21,22] All of these provocative tests can result in false-positive and false-negative results.

All patients need a dilated fundus examination as part of their work up. The mydriatic provocative test can be performed as part of the routine clinical examination when gonioscopy is equivocal. In patients where the angle is clearly almost occluded it is prudent to carry out prophylactic LPI before dilating the pupil. In a patient where the angle appearance is not so clear cut, i.e. they have a narrow angle without signs of angle closure or PAS, a short-acting mydriatic such as tropicamide can be instilled in one of their eyes. It is inadvisable to try this in both eyes as it may trigger a bilateral AAC, and it is sensible to avoid sympathomimetics, such as phenylephrine, as it can make any attack harder to abort. IOP and gonioscopy should be repeated approximately 30–60 minutes after the mydriatic is instilled. If the IOP is elevated by more than 5 mmHg and gonioscopy shows a closed or narrower angle than before dilatation, the test should be considered positive and an LPI planned.

Some patients have a pressure rise after dilatation anyway, particularly patients with PDS. It is important that any IOP rise is confirmed to be related to angle changes by repeat gonioscopy. Slit lamp examination may pick up the presence of pigment in the AC which could be the causative factor in any IOP spike detected.

Any angle closure attack induced by mydriasis should be treated aggressively as outlined earlier. As previously stated the greatest risk occurs when the pupil is returning to normal and lingers in the mid-dilated position, thus maximizing pupil block.

Treatment is not without risks and, as with every intervention, the risk versus benefit profile should be assessed. Without treatment occludable angles or patients suspected of PAC may progress to AACG (i.e. develop IOP-related glaucomatous visual-field defects) at a rate of 22% over the following 5 years.[23]

LPI should be carried out if:

- There is a history of or clinical evidence of subacute angle closure attacks
- There are any PAS in the angle related to appositional angle closure
- The trabecular meshwork is not visible for more than 270°
- The angles are potentially but not definitively occludable and the patient is likely to have difficulty accessing medical care should they develop an AAC attack. Patients just about to go on a 3-month expedition to the Amazon may elect to have prophylactic treatment than take the chance of running into difficulty days away from appropriate medical facilities

Prognosis and follow-up

Even after an apparently successful LPI has been performed the patient is still at risk of problems:

(1) The LPI may not actually be full thickness and the patient may still develop pupil block and AAC.
(2) A significant number of PAC patients will require IOP-lowering treatment despite apparent opening of the angle after LPI. Patients may have a mixed mechanism for their glaucoma. The previous attacks of AAC may have resulted in TM dysfunction.
(3) The patient may actually have a plateau iris syndrome rather than pupil block as a cause for their AAC.

All PAC patients should be considered glaucoma suspects for life and receive appropriate follow-up care. IOP measurements should be taken regularly and there should be regular assessment of the optic nerve and visual field. At each visit patency of the iridotomy should be assessed and gonioscopy should be ideally repeated. It must be remembered that the lens continues to grow throughout life and thus the angle may become narrower over time.

References

1. Van Herick W, Schaffer RN, Schwartz A. Estimation of width of angle of anterior chamber. Incidence and significance of the narrow angle. Am J Ophthalmol 1969; 68: 626.
2. Cockburn DM. Slit-lamp estimate of anterior chamber depth as a predictor of the gonioscopic visibility of the angle structures. Am J Optom Physiol Opt 1982; 59: 904.
3. Congdon N, Wang F, Tielsch JM. Issues in the epidemiology and population-based screening of primary angle-closure glaucoma. Surv Ophthalmol 1992; 36: 411.
4. Alsbirk PH. Primary angle-closure glaucoma: oculometry, epidemiology and genetics in a high-risk population. Acta Ophthalmol 1976; 54: 5.
5. Cox JE. Angle-closure glaucoma among the Alaskan Eskimos. Glaucoma 1984; 6: 135.
6. He M, Foster PJ, Ge J, Huang W, Zheng Y, Friedman DS, Lee PS, Khaw PT. Prevalence and clinical characteristics of glaucoma in adult Chinese: a population-based study in Liwan District, Guangzhou. Invest Ophthalmol Vis Sci 2006; 47: 2782–2788.
7. Foster PJ. The epidemiology of primary angle closure and associated glaucomatous optic neuropathy. Semin Ophthalmol 2002; 17: 50–58.
8. Congdon N, Wang F, Tielsch JM. Issues in the epidemiology and population-based screening of primary angle-closure glaucoma. Surv Ophthalmol 1992; 36: 411.
9. Bengtsson B. The prevalence of glaucoma. Br J Ophthalmol 1981; 65: 46.
10. Garnias F, Mapstone R. Miotics in closed angle glaucoma. Br J Ophthalmol 1975; 59: 205.
11. Zimmerman T. Pilocarpine. Ophthalmology 1981; 88: 85.
12. Wollensak J, Zeisberg B. Pathophysiology, treatment, and prophylaxis of angle-closure glaucoma. Glaucoma 1986; 8: 3.
13. Greco JJ, Kelman CD. Systemic pilocarpine toxicity in the treatment of angle-closure glaucoma. Ann Ophthalmol 1973; 5: 57.
14. Hillman J. Management of acute glaucoma with pilocarpine-soaked hydrophilic lens. Br J Ophthalmol 1974; 58: 674.
15. Iwata K, Abe H, Sugiyama J. Argon laser iridotomy in primary angle-closure glaucoma. Glaucoma 1985; 7: 103.
16. Lim LS, Aung T, Husain R, Wu YJ, Gazzard G, Seah SK. Acute primary angle closure: configuration of the drainage angle in the first year after laser peripheral iridotomy. Ophthalmology 2004; 111: 1470–1474.
17. Etter JR, Affel EL, Rhee DJ. High prevalence of plateau iris configuration in family members of patients with plateau iris syndrome. J Glaucoma 2006; 15: 394–398.
18. Ritch R, Tham CC, Lam DS. Long-term success of argon laser peripheral iridoplasty in the management of plateau iris syndrome. Ophthalmology 2004; 111: 104–108.
19. Lai JS, Tham CC, Chua JK, Poon AS, Lam DS. Laser peripheral iridoplasty as initial treatment of acute attack of primary angle-closure: a long-term follow-up study. J Glaucoma 2002; 11: 484–487.
20. Foster PJ, Aung T, Nolan WP, *et al.* Defining 'occludable' angles in population surveys: drainage angle width, peripheral anterior synechiae, and glaucomatous optic neuropathy in east Asian people. Br J Ophthalmol 2004; 88: 486–490.

21. American Academy of Ophthalmology. Preferred Practice Pattern. Primary Angle-Closure Glaucoma. San Francisco: American Academy of Ophthalmology 1992.
22. Ritch R. Definitive signs and gonioscopic visualization of appositional angle closure are indications for prophylactic laser iridectomy. Surv Ophthalmol 1996; 41: 31.
23. Thomas R, George R, Parikh R, Muliyil J, Jacob A. Five year risk of progression of primary angle closure suspects to primary angle closure: a population based study. Br J Ophthalmol 2003; 87: 450–454.

Chapter 23

Secondary angle closure

Secondary angle closure (SAC) describes a spectrum of conditions which all lead to closure of the drainage angle, usually by development of a fibrovascular membrane or scar tissue. The angle in these patients starts off open and then gradually closes off due to the underlying systemic or ocular pathology.

As in the assessment of PAC, examination of the fellow eye is key in the diagnostic process. The fellow eye (assuming it is unaffected) should not have features consistent with a narrow occludable angle.

SAC is divided into two groups:

(1) Where pupil block occurs
(2) Where no pupil block occurs

In the latter group when no pupil block occurs the pathology may be due to conditions that cause a direct physical obstruction of the trabecular meshwork (TM), such as angle neovascularization or PAS formation, and those that cause forward displacement of the ciliary body, for example as a result of ciliochoroidal effusion in the posterior segment.

Secondary angle-closure glaucoma (SACG) is distinct from SAC because in the former the raised IOP has resulted in glaucomatous optic neuropathy.

Clinically the eye is usually painful and red with reduced visual acuity. Gonioscopy should confirm the cause of the angle obstruction. The clinician will be able to detect the presence of PAS or the fibrovascular membrane associated with neovascularization of the angle. Slit lamp examination will reveal the presence of posterior synechiae and iris bombé if that is the etiology of the angle closure. A closed angle necessitates examination of the other eye. If that eye also has a similarly narrow angle then PAC is the likely diagnosis (unless that eye also suffers from the same disorder of course). If the other angle is open then a SAC is the likely culprit.

Management of SAC/SACG varies according to the underlying etiology, the IOP, the degree of glaucoma caused and the mechanism of angle closure. Medical management is instituted immediately to lower the IOP. Once the IOP has been reduced, the mechanism of angle closure must be identified and addressed appropriately.

Secondary angle closure with pupillary block

Underlying etiologies of secondary angle closure

Underlying etiologies include:

- With pupillary block:
  - Phacomorphic glaucoma
  - Lens subluxation/ectopia lentis
  - Pseudophakic and aphakic pupillary block
  - Inflammation with 360° posterior synechiae
- Without pupillary block – direct obstruction of the trabecular meshwork:
  - Neovascular glaucoma
  - Iridocorneal endothelial syndrome
  - PAS secondary to inflammation
- Without pupillary block – forward displacement of ciliary body:
  - Ciliary block (malignant) glaucoma
  - Cysts of the iris or ciliary body
  - Intraocular neoplasm
  - Ciliochoroidal effusion
  - Inflammatory: scleritis, pars planitis
  - Uveal effusion syndrome (idiopathic)
  - After scleral buckling surgery
  - Suprachoroidal hemorrhage

Phacomorphic glaucoma

In this condition the cataractous lens is implicated in the anterior displacement of the iris and the angle closure. It is probably a form of PAC as the patient has an anatomically predisposed angle which is tipped over the edge into closure by the progressive swelling of the cataractous lens. If the angle of the other eye is open, however, we can rest the blame squarely on the cataract and make a diagnosis of true phacomorphic glaucoma.

In phacomorphic glaucoma, after the acute attack is reversed, surgical intervention is usually necessary. LPI will reverse the pupillary block, but cataract surgery is usually the definitive treatment for the glaucoma and also results in visual improvement.

Lens subluxation/ectopia lentis

Ectopia lentis describes the condition whereby a lens is completely or incompletely dislocated. A subluxated lens remains behind the iris but is loose as a result of laxity or breakage of the supporting zonules. If the lens moves forward it can result in a pupil block or displacement of the peripheral iris forward and subsequent angle closure. Ectopia lentis can be secondary to trauma, ocular disease or certain hereditary conditions such as Marfan's syndrome.

Inflammation with 360° posterior synechiae

Pupillary block glaucoma may follow severe cases of uveitis if 360° of posterior synechiae form, resulting in no communication between the posterior and anterior chambers with iris bombé and AAC. This form of pupillary block glaucoma should be treated quickly and aggressively to break the posterior synechiae and stop formation of PAS which leads to permanent and irreversible angle closure. If the posterior synechiae cannot be released a peripheral iridotomy is required.

Neovascular glaucoma

Established angle neovascularization leads to irreversible angle closure which often leads to severe glaucoma. It is frequently very difficult to treat with a reasonably poor prognosis for IOP control. If the angle neovascularization is picked up early and the underlying condition is treated we can prevent the formation of the permanent fibrovascular membrane which permanently blocks off the angle and causes the chronic IOP rise. Therefore, early diagnosis of iris or angle neovascularization, with prompt and aggressive treatment, is warranted to try to preserve vision.

Neovascularization of the iris and angle primarily result from hypoxic retinal conditions, the most common being central retinal vein occlusion (CRVO), diabetic retinopathy (DR) and ocular ischemic syndrome. Although the underlying etiology of neovascularization may vary, the pathogenesis of angle obstruction and the clinical appearance of the angle are similar.

The severity and extent of retinal ischemia fuels the rapidity of onset of anterior segment neovascularization to different degrees. For example, angle neovascularization associated with an ischemic CRVO may develop in a few weeks and often within the first 90 days after the acute event (hence the classical description of 90-day glaucoma).

Neovascularization is stimulated by the release of angiogenic factors from hypoxic retinal tissue. The new vessels usually begin at the pupil margin, enlarge and grow in an irregular pattern along the iris surface. The vessels are accompanied by a fibrous membrane which is actually the entity that causes the problem. This fibrovascular membrane grows towards the angle and then eventually over the TM resulting in partial obstruction of aqueous outflow. The membrane eventually contracts and pulls the peripheral iris on to the TM, leading to the formation of PAS and complete blockage of the trabeculum. This process of contraction may pull the anterior iris tissue radially, causing the pigmented layer of the iris to prolapse and roll forwards resulting in ectropion uvea.

Patients with any of the conditions in Box 23.1 should undergo careful high-magnification slit lamp examination of the iris at each visit with the specific purpose of identifying the presence of new vessel growth. In addition patients who have had a CRVO or who have severe non-proliferative or proliferative diabetic retinopathy should have gonioscopy at every follow-up visit to detect the early onset of any angle neovascularization.

Presentation depends upon how far down the pathological process the patient is. If early, the eye may be quiet with no signs of inflammation or injection. The only signs may be a slightly raised IOP and fine new vessels at the pupil margin and within the angle. The condition is potentially reversible at this stage with aggressive treatment of the underlying disorder. Pan-retinal photocoagulation (PRP) should be performed at the first sign of iris or angle

Box 23.1 Causes of neovascular glaucoma.

Ocular vascular disease
Central or branch retinal vein occlusion
Central or branch retinal artery occlusion
Diabetic retinopathy
Carotid artery disease/insufficiency
Retinal detachment particularly if chronic
Sickle cell retinopathy
Ocular neoplasms
Chronic uveitis
Endophthalmitis
Sympathetic ophthalmia

neovascularization. After adequate and prompt PRP, the angle vessels can begin to regress within days. Additional fill-in PRP sessions may be required if the neovascularization fails to reverse. The IOP may come back down to normal or anti-glaucoma medication may still be needed, despite opening of the angle, to treat residual TM dysfunction.

With further progression the fibrovascular membrane within the angle matures and causes the formation of PAS with a significant rise in IOP. At this stage treating the underlying ischemic process will not cause reversal of the SAC and all efforts should be directed at IOP control. Patients usually present with a red eye with evidence of corneal edema, AC cellular reaction and sometimes a hyphema. At this stage the iris and angle neovascularization are usually obvious, assuming the cornea is clear enough to allow an adequate view.

Trabeculectomy may be required, however it is at high risk of failure. A glaucoma drainage device (GDD) may be required in such cases. If all useful vision is lost all attempts should be directed at keeping the eye comfortable and maintaining an adequate cosmetic appearance. Cyclodiode laser is usually effective to control IOP. The chronic use of cycloplegics (such as atropine 1%) and topical steroids may ensure comfort is maintained long term.

Iridocorneal endothelial syndrome

Iridocorneal endothelial (ICE) syndrome describes a spectrum of disorders with a common pathology arising from uncontrolled and pathological growth of corneal endothelial cells. It is usually unilateral, non-hereditary and more common in women than in men.

The ICE syndromes are progressive iris atrophy, Chandler syndrome and Cogan-Reese (iris naevus) syndrome. They are essentially all part of the same disorder but each has a different prominent feature. Progressive iris atrophy manifests as iris holes and PAS. Chandler syndrome is the most common variant and manifests as corneal abnormalities. It is characterized by a fine beaten-silver appearance to the corneal endothelium, and corneal edema is an early and prominent sign. Cogan-Reese (iris naevus) syndrome shows as the presence of numerous pigmented iris nodules.

Common to all of the ICE syndromes is the underlying disorder of the corneal endothelium. The endothelium is dysfunctional and corneal edema with blurred vision may ensue (seen more in the Chandler syndrome). If the corneal endothelium grows out as a membrane across the angle, PAS form and the angle is blocked with subsequent raised IOP. Contraction of this membrane may lead to progressive synechial angle closure, corectopia, ectropion uvea, iris atrophy and iris hole formation.

Patients with SAC secondary to ICE syndrome present with pain, decreased vision and iris abnormalities. The pain and decreased acuity may be a result of the corneal edema or the elevated IOP.

The prognosis in these cases is not great. Trabeculectomies tend to fail eventually due to growth of the ICE membrane into the scleral flap thus closing it off. GDDs can work for a period but again are prone to failure. The saving grace of this condition is that it is unilateral and the other eye is normal.

SAC due to uveitis and inflammatory conditions

Surgery, trauma and idiopathic or specific inflammatory conditions (for example sarcoidosis or ankylosing spondylitis) can lead to SAC through the deposition of inflammatory cells and debris in the angle with PAS formation. Signs of previous or current intraocular inflammation are usually evident and gonioscopy usually reveals obvious PAS with no view of normal TM.

Management involves suppressing the inflammation and the use of anti-glaucoma medication. Miotics are contraindicated because they induce ciliary spasm, increase inflammation and predispose to the formation of posterior synechiae. Topical prostaglandins should be avoided because they can exacerbate the inflammatory component.

The use of steroids to suppress the inflammation may be problematic as they themselves may induce a steroid response contributing or even solely responsible for the raised IOP. Rimexolone (Vexol) may be useful in such cases because it has a potency similar to that of prednisolone acetate but is less prone to stimulating a steroid response. Steroid-sparing agents such as topical non-steroidal anti-inflammatory drops may be helpful in suppressing the uveitis without causing an iatrogenic IOP rise.

Trabeculectomy is high risk in these cases and anti-metabolites should be used to maximize success. All active inflammation should be suppressed optimally before surgery is contemplated. Prophylactic systemic steroids may be appropriate to minimize peri- and post-operative inflammation in these cases.

Ciliary block glaucoma

Ciliary block glaucoma, also known as malignant glaucoma, is a rare type of SAC that is usually seen as a complication of intraocular surgery for angle-closure glaucoma. The term malignant glaucoma was coined because of the poor prognosis and unsatisfactory response to medical treatment in patients with this disease. It has also been reported to occur after Nd:YAG capsulotomy, laser iridotomy and cataract or filtering surgery, and it has occurred spontaneously and after trauma, inflammation, the use of miotics and exfoliation syndrome.

Ciliary block glaucoma occurs in an anatomically predisposed eye that has a decreased space between the ciliary body and the adjacent lens. This may exist in several situations, including an eye with a smaller globe and normal-sized lens (nanophthalmos), increased lens size caused by an aging or cataract formation, a decrease in the anterior–posterior lens position as the result of weakened or slackened zonules (e.g. secondary to pseudoexfoliation of the lens capsule or trauma), or after contraction or swelling of the ciliary body (e.g. caused by inflammation or vascular engorgement). These predisposing anatomical considerations facilitate the formation of a seal between the anterior hyaloid and the ciliary body.

This apposition prevents the usual flow of aqueous from posterior chamber to anterior chamber. Flow is pathologically directed posteriorly into the vitreous space. As the aqueous is pumped into the vitreous cavity the posterior segment pressure increases and the lens and iris are pushed forwards causing shallowing of the AC.

Ciliary block glaucoma occurs immediately to months after ocular surgery (e.g. cataract extraction or filtering surgery).

Examination reveals central and peripheral shallowing of the AC along with a mild to moderately elevated IOP. A peripheral iridotomy can be present and patent in this condition as the hyaloid face, not the iris, is the structure preventing normal anterior flow of aqueous.

Medical treatment is tried initially with mydriatic–cycloplegic agents (atropine and phenylephrine) and topical ocular hypotensive agents. If the IOP fails to respond oral or systemic hyperosmotic agents may be used.

If the attack cannot be reversed then laser (either argon or Nd:YAG) can be applied to the anterior hyaloid face to try and create a break in it, and thus allow flow of the trapped aqueous into the anterior chamber.

If medical and laser treatment fail to resolve the attack then surgical treatment with the aim of creating a defect in the anterior hyaloid face is required. Surgical aspiration of vitreous or anterior vitrectomy may be performed to reverse the ciliary block.

Chapter 24

Steroid-induced glaucoma

It is a well recognized fact that some patients will experience a significant rise in IOP with the use of topical, intraocular, periocular or systemic corticosteroids. In many cases the condition is reversible, however in some the pressure elevation can be chronic and result in glaucomatous optic neuropathy (steroid-induced glaucoma). This pressure rise occurs more commonly in individuals who have chronic open-angle glaucoma (COAG) or a family history of the disease.

Approximately 18–36% of the general population are corticosteroid responders.[1] This response is increased to 46–92% in patients with primary open-angle glaucoma (POAG).[1] Patients over 40 years of age and with certain systemic diseases (e.g. diabetes mellitus, high myopia) as well as relatives of patients with POAG are more vulnerable to corticosteroid-induced glaucoma.

Steroid response is most commonly identified as a complication of topical steroid use with drugs such as dexamethasone or prednisolone. In responsive patients, the IOP typically rises after several weeks of continual treatment and in most individuals it returns to normal following cessation of therapy.

Factors contributing to steroid response

Glaucoma/glaucoma suspects

Back in the 1960s, research[2] demonstrated that patients who had glaucoma or were deemed glaucoma suspects, sustained a marked rise in IOP in response to several weeks of exposure to topical corticosteroids. The IOP for the glaucoma group rose from a mean of 16.9 mmHg to 32.1 mmHg and that for the glaucoma suspect group rose from a mean of 17.1 mmHg to 28.3 mmHg. In their normal group some patients experienced no IOP rise while another group experienced a moderate IOP increase. Overall the mean IOP increased from 13.6 to only 18.2 mmHg in the normals. The IOP for all the patients they studied returned to their baseline or to a normal level after cessation of the steroid treatment. It is thus clear that patients may have a greater risk of experiencing an IOP increase if they are known to or suspected of having glaucoma.

Age

Armaly[3,4] has reported that the steroid-induced ocular hypertension occurs to a greater extent in older compared with younger eyes.

Family history

Patients with a first-degree relative with POAG are at greater risk of suffering a significant pressure increase with corticosteroid administration.[5–7]

Methods of administration

A steroid response has been seen associated with both topical and systemic administration of corticosteroid.

Topical therapy

Topical corticosteroid therapy is more often associated with an IOP rise than is the case with systemic administration. This may occur with drops or ointment applied directly to the eye and with steroid preparations used in treating the skin of the eyelids.[8,9]

Periocular therapy

Periocular injection of a long-acting corticosteroid has a significant chance of producing troublesome steroid-induced ocular hypertension. IOP elevation may occur in response to subconjunctival, subtenon, or retrobulbar injections of steroids.[10–13] Unfortunately the lack of a previous steroid response to topical steroids does not mean that an individual will have no steroid response to periocular corticosteroids.[12] Depot steroids are dangerous because of their prolonged duration of action, and their lack of accessibility once placed into the orbit. Sometimes surgical exploration and excision is required.[14]

Intravitreal therapy

Intravitreal steroids can also cause a rise in IOP. Injection of triamcinolone acetonide in an attempt to treat intraocular neovascular or inflammatory diseases can raise the IOP by several mmHg in most patients treated within 3–4 weeks of initiating treatment.[15–17] The use of this treatment is increasing in popularity as is the likelihood of us facing pressure problems related to it. (See intravitreal triamcinolone below.)

Systemic therapy

Systemic administration of corticosteroids is least likely to induce glaucoma, although cases have been described.[18-22] In one study of 62 patients receiving systemic steroids after renal transplantation, six developed IOP.[22] IOP elevation has been associated with inhaled and nasal corticosteroids[23,24], and it has been reported that amounts of corticosteroids sufficient to cause an IOP elevation can be absorbed from dermatological application in areas away from the eyes.[25]

In one study[26] users of nasal corticosteroids were shown to be at increased risk of ocular hypertension or glaucoma with an odds ratio of 1.44, possibly due to a mechanism related to chronic steroid use.

Intravitreal triamcinolone

Recently, the use of intraocular steroid injection has become more popular as a treatment modality for many medical retina conditions. Fortunately, although it has been shown that depot intravitreal administration of triamcinolone can produce IOP rises,[27] the majority of affected patients have been controlled with topical ocular hypotensive therapy. Some patients, however, develop intractable glaucoma which may require surgical intervention.[28]

One study[29] investigated 12 patients who demonstrated a steroid response to injected corticosteroid and showed that the duration and severity of response was inversely related to preparation solubility. Interestingly most of these patients had been previously treated with topical steroids without any pressure response. This data again suggests that lack of IOP change with topical steroid use cannot predict the IOP response with depot steroid injections.

A further study[30] looked at more than 500 patients having intravitreal triamcinolone at a dose of 4 mg/0.1 ml. More than 50% had an IOP elevation of at least 30% while 14.2% had an increase in IOP of 10 mmHg or more. Baseline IOP greater than 16 mmHg was a risk factor for post-injection IOP elevation.

In another study[31] 40.4% experienced a pressure elevation to 24 mmHg or higher at a mean of 100.6 days after treatment. Of non-glaucomatous patients with a baseline IOP of 15 mmHg or above, 60.0% experienced a pressure elevation, compared with only 22.7% of those with a baseline pressure below 15 mmHg. In glaucoma patients, 6 of 12 (50%) experienced a pressure elevation, and this elevation was not correlated with baseline pressure.

Different preparations

The potency of the corticosteroid used tends to correlate with the potential steroid response it can induce. Dexamethasone and prednisolone are commonly used, potent corticosteroids with a significant tendency to trigger an ocular hypertensive steroid-response.

Cantrill and colleagues[32] have published data on the level of steroid response in known high responders to steroids of different potencies (Table 24.1).

Table 24.1 IOP elevations for different steroid preparations.

Preparation	Average pressure rise (mmHg)
Dexamethasone 0.1%	22.0 ± 2.9
Prednisolone 1.0%	10.0 ± 1.7
Dexamethasone 0.005%	8.2 ± 1.7
Fluorometholone 0.1%	6.1 ± 1.4
Hydrocortisone 0.5%	3.2 ± 1.0
Tetrahydrotriamcinolone 0.25%	1.8 ± 1.3
Medrysone 1.0%	1.0 ± 1.3

Suggested mechanisms of the corticosteroid response

Corticosteroids are believed to decrease outflow by inhibiting degradation of extracellular matrix material in the trabecular meshwork (TM), leading to aggregation of an excessive amount of the material within the outflow channels and a subsequent increase in outflow resistance.[33-35] Several researchers[36,37] suggested that this response might be due to an alteration of the metabolism of mucopolysaccharides, leading to their accumulation in the TM.

In addition to the above, corticosteroids also decrease the phagocytic properties of TM cells. These cells filter and clear debris from the aqueous before it enters Schlemm's canal. Steroid-induced inhibition of this process could result in accumulation of debris and increased resistance to outflow.

Structural changes in the TM cells have also been proposed as a part of the pathogenesis of this phenomenon.[38,39] One group of researchers[39] discovered that dexamethasone caused cross-linkage of actin fibers, leading to the formation of networks within cultured human TM cells and went on to document an IOP increase in steroid-treated, perfusion-cultured human eyes.[40]

The different theories described above emphasize that this condition is not fully understood. The likelihood is that all of the above changes contribute to the increased aqueous ouflow resistance seen.

Clinical aspects

The clinical characteristics of corticosteroid-induced glaucoma are the same as those for POAG, except that patients have a history of corticosteroid use.

Prevention is better than cure and so the clinician should maintain an index of suspicion in eyes treated with topical, periocular or intraocular steroids and follow them up appropriately with regular IOP assessments. Steroids should be used with caution in patients with glaucoma or a positive family history of glaucoma. In patients at risk of a significant IOP rise it is prudent to avoid depot injections, as should a steroid response occur the removal of the steroid is difficult.

The insidious nature of this condition requires careful monitoring of patients at risk to identify any early pressure increase that would necessitate either withdrawal of steroid or the commencement of anti-glaucoma medications. A baseline measurement of IOP should be taken prior to commencement of any corticosteroid therapy. Patients on topical therapy should have their

IOP measured a few weeks after commencement of treatment and then at regular intervals thereafter until the steroids are discontinued. Patients having intravitreal steroid injections should be monitored for several months following their steroid injection. It is prudent to advise patients on long-term systemic steroid therapy that they should attend their own optician for a regular IOP check.

If an IOP rise is detected the risk–benefit of continuation of steroid therapy should be judged. If the benefits outweigh the risks then anti-glaucoma medication should be considered to temporarily reduce IOP until the steroid treatment can be stopped. The steroid response usually resolves in 1–4 weeks.[41]

If the need for anti-inflammatory medication is great then there are alternatives to potent corticosteroid use. The treatment can be changed to preparations such as fluorometholone 0.1% or rimexolone 1%, which are claimed to have less effect on IOP.[42] In certain situations non-steroidal anti-inflammatory drugs (NSAIDs) may be used as 'steroid-sparing' agents.

In about 3% of cases this steroid response may be irreversible.[43] This is a particular risk when there is a family history of glaucoma or long-term chronic use of steroid.

Medical treatment is the first line however some patients may require a trabeculectomy if the IOP cannot be controlled.

When faced with a patient who sustains an IOP rise after a depot injection which is not controlled medically, excision of the depot steroid may be required. With the increasing popularity of intravitreal triamcinolone injections,[44,45] vitrectomy may prove useful in preventing glaucoma in selected cases.

References

1. Tripathi RC, Parapuram SK, Tripathi BJ, Zhong Y, Chalam KV. Corticosteroids and glaucoma risk. Drugs Aging 1999; 15: 439–450.
2. Becker B, Mills DW. Corticosteroids and intraocular pressure. Arch Ophthalmol 1963; 70: 500–507.
3. Armaly MF. Effect of corticosteroids on intraocular pressure and fluid dynamics: I. The effect of dexamethasone in the normal eye. Arch Ophthalmol 1963; 70: 482–491.
4. Armaly MF. Effect of corticosteroids on intraocular pressure and fluid dynamics: II. The effect of dexamethasone on the glaucomatous eye. Arch Ophthalmol 1963; 70: 492–499.
5. Becker B. Intraocular pressure response to topical corticosteroids. Invest Ophthalmol 1965; 26: 198–205.
6. Becker B, Hahn KA. Topical corticosteroids and heredity in primary open-angle glaucoma. Am J Ophthalmol 1964; 54: 543–551.
7. Davies TG. Tonographic survey of the close relatives of patients with chronic simple glaucoma. Br J Ophthalmol 1968; 52: 32–39.
8. Cubey RB. Glaucoma following the application of corticosteroid to the skin of the eyelids. Br J Dermatol 1976; 95: 207.
9. Zugerman C, Sanders D, Levit F. Glaucoma from topically applied steroids. Arch Dermatol 1976; 112: 1326.
10. Kalina RE. Increased intraocular pressure following subconjunctival corticosteroid administration. Arch Ophthalmol 1969; 81: 788.
11. Herschler J. Intractable intraocular hypertension induced by repository triamcinolone acetonide. Am J Ophthalmol 1972; 74: 501.

12. Herschler J. Increased intraocular pressure induced by repository corticosteroids. Am J Ophthalmol 1976; 82: 90.
13. Ferry AP, Harris WP, Nelson MH. Histopathologic features of subconjunctivally injected corticosteroids. Am J Ophthalmol 1987; 103: 716.
14. Akduman L, Kolker AE, Black DL, *et al.* Treatment of persistent glaucoma secondary to periocular corticosteroids. Am J Ophthalmol 1996; 122: 275.
15. Wingate RJ, Beaumont PE. Intravitreal triamcinolone and elevated intraocular pressure. Aust N Z J Ophthalmol 1999; 27: 431.
16. Bakri SJ, Beer PM. The effect of intravitreal triamcinolone acetonide on intraocular pressure. Ophth Surg Lasers Imaging 2003; 34: 386.
17. Jonas JB, Kreissig I, Degenring R. Intraocular pressure after intravitreal injection of triamcinolone acetonide. Br J Ophthalmol 2003; 87: 24.
18. Stern JJ. Acute glaucoma during cortisone therapy. Am J Ophthalmol 1953; 36: 389.
19. Covell LL. Glaucoma induced by systemic steroid therapy. Am J Ophthalmol 1958; 45: 108.
20. Godel V, Feiler-Ofry V, Stein R. Systemic steroids and ocular fluid dynamics. I. Analysis of the sample as a whole: influence of dosage and duration of therapy. Acta Ophthalmol 1972; 50: 655.
21. Godel V, Feiler-Ofry V, Stein R. Systemic steroids and ocular fluid dynamics. II. Systemic versus topical steroids. Acta Ophthalmol 1972; 50: 664.
22. Adhikary HP, Sells RA, Basu PK. Ocular complications of systemic steroid after renal transplantation and their association with HLA. Br J Ophthalmol 1982; 66: 290.
23. Opatowsky I, Feldman RM, Gross R, *et al.* Intraocular pressure elevation associated with inhalation and nasal corticosteroids. Ophthalmology 1995; 102: 177.
24. Schwartzenberg GW, Buys YM. Glaucoma secondary to topical use of steroid cream. Can J Ophthalmol 1999; 34: 222.
25. Mitchell P, Gumming RG, Mackey DA. Inhaled corticosteroids, family history, and risk of glaucoma. Ophthalmology 1999; 106: 2301.
26. Garbe E, Lorier J, Boivin JF, Siussa S. Inhaled and nasal glucocorticoids and the risk of ocular hypertension or open-angle glaucoma. JAMA 1997; 277: 722–727.
27. Gillies MC, Simpson JM, Billson FA, Luo W, Penfold P, Chua W, *et al.* Safety of an intravitreal injection of triamcinolone: results from a randomized clinical trial. Arch Ophthalmol 2004; 122: 336–340.
28. Kaushik S, Gupta V, Gupta A, Dogra MR, Singh R. Intractable glaucoma following intravitreal triamcinolone in central retinal vein occlusion. Am J Ophthalmol 2004; 137: 758–760.
29. Herschler J. Increased intraocular pressure induced by repository corticosteroids. Am J Ophthalmol 1976; 82: 90–93.
30. Rhee DJ, Peck RE, Belmont J, Martidis A, Liu M, Chang J, Fontanarosa J, Moster MR. Intraocular pressure alterations following intravitreal triamcinolone acetonide. Br J Ophthalmol. 2006; 90: 999–1003.
31. Smithen LM, Ober MD, Maranan L, Spaide RF. Intravitreal triamcinolone acetonide and intraocular pressure. Am J Ophthalmol 2004; 138: 740–743.
32. Cantrill HL, Palmberg, Zink HA, Waltman SR, Podos SM, Becker B. Comparison of *in vitro* potency of corticosteroids with ability to raise intraocular pressure. Am J Ophthalmol 1975; 79: 1012–1017.
33. Renfro L, Snow JS. Ocular effects of topical and systemic steroids. Dermatol Clin 1992; 10: 505–510.
34. Wordinger RJ, Clark AF. Effects of glucocorticoids on the trabecular meshwork: towards a better understanding of glaucoma. 34. Prog Retina Eye Res 1999; 18: 629–667.
35. Jones R 3rd, Rhee DJ. Corticosteroid-induced ocular hypertension and glaucoma: a brief review and update of the literature. Curr Opin Ophthalmol 2006; 17: 163–167.
36. Francois J. Corticosteroid glaucoma. Ann Ophthalmol 1977; 9: 1075–1080.

37. Armaly MF. Effect of corticosteroids on intraocular pressure and fluid dynamics: I. The effect of dexamethasone in the normal eye. Arch Ophthalmol 1963; 70: 482–491.
38. Tripathi BJ, Tripathi RC, Swift HH. Hydrocortisone-induced DNA endoreplication in human trabecular cell *in vitro*. Exp Eye Res 1989; 49: 259–270.
39. Clark AF, Wilson K, McCartney MD, Miggans ST, Kunkle M, Howe W. Glucocorticoid-induced formation of cross-linked actin networks in cultured human trabecular meshwork cells. Invest Ophthamol Vis Sci 1994; 35: 281–294.
40. Clark AF, Wilson K, de Kater AW, Allingham R, McCartney MD. Dexamethasone-induced ocular hypertension in perfusion-cultured human eyes. Invest Ophthalmol Vis Sci 1995; 36: 478–489.
41. Weinreb RN, Polansky JR, Kramer SG, BaxterJD. Acute effects of dexamethasone on intraocular pressure in glaucoma. Invest Ophthalmol Vis Sci 1985; 26: 170–175.
42. Cantrill HL, Palmberg, Zink HA, Waltman SR, Podos SM, Becker B. Comparison of *in vitro* potency of corticosteroids with ability to raise intraocular pressure. Am J Ophthalmol 1975; 79: 1012–1017.
43. Francois J. Corticosteroid glaucoma. Ann Ophthalmol 1977; 9: 1075–1080.
44. Chen SD, Lochhead J, Patel CK, Frith P. Intravitreal triamcinolone acetonide for ischaemic macular oedema caused by branch retinal vein occlusion. Br J Ophthalmol 2004; 88: 154–155.
45. Spaide RF, Sorenson J, Maranan L. Combined photodynamic therapy with verteporfin and intravitreal triamcinolone acetonide for choroidal neovascularization. Ophthamology 2003; 110: 1517–1525.

Chapter 25

Landmark studies

The Ocular Hypertension Treatment Study (OHTS)[1]

This study was designed to determine whether topical hypotensive medication can delay or prevent the onset of primary open-angle glaucoma (POAG) in patients with ocular hypertension.

This was a five-year multicentre randomized controlled trial. More than 1500 patients with ocular hypertension (no evidence of glaucoma damage and IOPs ranging from 24–32 mmHg in one eye and 21–32 mmHg in the other) were randomized to treatment or no treatment. Drops were selected and changed by the clinician in order to achieve a target IOP of less than 24 mmHg and at least a 20% reduction in IOP from baseline. The end-point was progression to POAG defined as the development of a reproducible glaucomatous visual-field defect or optic disc deterioration consistent with POAG.

Over the course of the study, the mean IOP reduction in the treated group was 22.5 ± 9.9% compared to 4 ± 11.6% in the untreated group. In the treated group 4.4% of the patients developed glaucoma while in the untreated group 9.5% developed glaucoma. Therefore treatment reduced the risk of progressing to glaucoma by half.

Key clinical points

- In OHT patients topical treatment was effective in delaying or preventing the onset of POAG.
- For patients with moderate to high risk of developing POAG, IOP-lowering treatment should be considered.
- Good predictors for developing POAG were found to be: baseline IOP (the higher the greater the risk), age (older patients are more likely to get glaucoma), vertical CDR (the larger the cup the more likely the development of glaucoma).
- CCT was an independent risk factor for the development of glaucoma. The thinner the cornea the more likely the patient is to convert to glaucoma.
- The safety profile of treatment was good.

So what does this mean for us?

- Measure CCT in all OHT patients.
- Patients with thinner corneas warrant consideration of treatment particularly if they have a higher IOP.
- In patients with thicker corneas it may be reasonable to simply observe them, obviously as long as their IOP isn't too high.
- Consider each case as an individual and take into account all the clinical findings before making a decision.

The Early Manifest Glaucoma Trial (EMGT)[2,3]

This trial aimed to compare the effect on progression of early-diagnosed open-angle glaucoma between two groups. One had immediate IOP-lowering treatment while the other had no treatment.

More than 250 patients with early diagnosed glaucoma (median IOP of 20 mmHg) were allocated at random to either trabeculoplasty plus hypotensive treatment (betaxolol) or no initial treatment and followed up for a median of 6 years. Glaucoma progression was defined by specific visual field and/or optic disc evidence of worsening parameters. This judgment was based upon serial tonometry, optic disc examination, regular 3-monthly visual fields and optic disc photographs every 6 months.

Early treatment to lower IOP had a markedly beneficial effect on outcome. The average sustained IOP reduction was 5.1 mmHg (25%) from baseline in the treated group. The relative risk of disease progression was 27.4% lower in the treated group. When disease progression did occur, early treatment delayed progression by a median of 18 months compared to controls (66 months to progression in the treated group versus 48 months in those not on any treatment).

Key clinical points

- The study showed that in early glaucoma, lowering IOP produced a 27.4% reduction in the relative risk of glaucoma progression.
- For each 1 mmHg of IOP reduction there was an estimated 10% decrease in risk of glaucoma progression.

So what does this mean for us?

- Lowering IOP in glaucoma patients is good.

The Collaborative Initial Glaucoma Treatment Study (CIGTS)[4]

This study assessed the effect of medical or surgical IOP lowering on early-diagnosed open-angle glaucoma patients. This is a prospective randomized multicentre trial, involving more than 600 patients. Patients were treated with either medication or surgery and evaluated 6-monthly for at least 4 years. The treatment was reasonably aggressive with the aim of reducing IOP to a predetermined target level customized for the individual patient. Progression of disease was assessed primarily though visual field loss, with visual acuity, IOP and cataract as secondary outcomes.

Initial surgical treatment achieved a reduction in IOP from a mean of 27 mmHg to around 14 mmHg. Corresponding reduction in the medication group was from a mean of 28 mmHg to around 17 mmHg. There was no significant difference in visual-field loss between the two groups. During follow-up, patients were at greater risk of visual acuity loss in the surgical group but by 4 years post-treatment both groups were comparable. The surgical group had a much higher rate of visually significant cataract formation.

Key clinical points

- Both medical treatment and surgery were equally effective in minimizing visual-field loss.
- It seems that the IOP lowering is the important factor.
- The surgical group had more complications.

So what does this mean for us?

- Lowering IOP in glaucoma patients is good.
- If we cannot lower the IOP to a satisfactory level by medical therapy we need to do surgery.

The Advanced Glaucoma Intervention Study (AGIS)[5]

This study assessed the role of IOP reduction in advanced glaucoma in preventing further glaucomatous field loss.

Almost 800 glaucoma eyes in almost 600 patients were randomly assigned to one of two groups. Half were randomized to argon laser trabeculoplasty (ALT) followed by filtering surgery while the other half had initial filtering surgery followed by ALT. If the patient had not achieved their target IOP or was progressing, the patient underwent a repeat trabeculectomy procedure. None of these glaucoma surgeries were performed with augmentation. In all patients attempts were made to reduce IOP to less than 18 mmHg. IOP and visual fields were assessed 6-monthly for a minimum of 6 years.

Patients with average IOP of less than 14 mmHg in the first 18 months of follow-up had very little change in visual defect score. The researchers looked at the IOPs at all the visits during follow-up. The group with an IOP of less than 18 mmHg at every follow-up visit showed virtually no change in mean visual defect score. These patients had a mean IOP of 12.3 mmHg over the whole duration of the study. All other groups showed significant worsening of visual fields. The more visits at which an IOP of more than 18 mmHg was recorded, the more likely the visual field was to worsen.

Key clinical points

- Keeping a patient's IOP at less than 18 mmHg over 6 years was associated with almost no visual-field loss. The average IOP for these eyes was low being 12.3 mmHg.
- Low post-intervention IOP is associated with reduced progression of visual defect.
- Achieving a low IOP early in this subset of severe glaucoma patients stabilized and prevented disease progression.

So what does this mean for us?

- We need to treat patients with advanced glaucoma aggressively to get their pressure down and keep it down consistently.
- Of course the risk versus benefit profile of the interventions should be considered and a frank discussion undertaken with the patient.

The Collaborative Normal-Tension Glaucoma Study (NTGS)[6]

This study looked at lowering IOP in normal-tension glaucoma (NTG). In a randomized prospective multicentre study, 140 patients/eyes with NTG (as defined by optic disc abnormalities and visual-field defects consistent with glaucoma but a measured IOP that never exceeded 24 mmHg) were randomized to two groups. Half were treated aggressively by medical and/or surgical intervention to lower IOP by 30% within 6 months and maintain it throughout the 4-year follow-up period. The second group were untreated controls. No patients were treated with beta-blockers or adrenergic agonists because of the potential cardiovascular, vasoconstrictive and crossover effects that could confound the data. Patients were monitored for visual-field progression or change in degree of glaucomatous optic disc damage.

Mean IOP levels during follow-up were 10.6 mm ± 2.7 mmHg in the treated group and 16.0 ± 2.1 mmHg in the untreated group. The proportion of eyes progressing was three times greater in the untreated group than in the treated group (35% vs 12%, $p < 0.05$).

Cataracts occurred more often in the treated group (38%) primarily in the surgically treated subgroup (26%). The proportion of cataracts occurring in the medically-treated subgroup (11%) was less than in the control group (14%) ($p = 0.00075$).

Key clinical points

- Glaucoma progression was seen in 35% of the control eyes versus 12% of the treated eyes.
- A 30% reduction in IOP slows the rate of progression of NTG.
- Interestingly despite these patients having previously demonstrated progression, 65% of untreated patients still did not show any progression during a follow-up period of 5 years or more.
- Additionally, 12% of the treated NTG patients continued to progress despite a 30% IOP reduction.

So what does this mean for us?

- Treating NTG patients seems to slow progression.
- But even if we don't treat them, 65% don't get worse anyway so maybe not everyone needs treatment.
- If the glaucoma is early it may be reasonable to observe the patient and then intervene and treat if they are actually getting worse.

References

1. Kass MA, Heuer DK, Higginbotham EJ, *et al*. The Ocular Hypertension Treatment Study: a randomized trial determines that topical ocular hypotensive medication delays or prevents the onset of primary open-angle glaucoma. Arch Ophthalmol 2002; 120: 701–713.
2. Heijl A, Leske C, Bengtsson B, *et al*. Reduction of intraocular pressure and glaucoma progression: results from the Early Manifest Glaucoma Trial. Arch Ophthalmol 2002; 120: 1268–1279.
3. Leske C, Heijl A, Hussein M, *et al*. Factors for glaucoma progression and the effect of treatment: the Early Manifest Glaucoma Trial. Arch Ophthalmol 2003; 121: 48–56.
4. Lichter P, Musch D, Gillespie B, *et al*. Interim clinical outcomes in the Collaborative Initial Glaucoma Treatment Study comparing initial treatment randomized to medications or surgery. Ophthalmology 2001; 108: 1943–1953.
5. The AGIS Investigators. The Advanced Glaucoma Intervention Study (AGIS): 7. The relationship between control of intraocular pressure and visual field deterioration. Am J of Ophthalmol 2000; 130: 429–440.
6. Collaborative Normal-Tension Glaucoma Study Group. Comparison of glaucomatous progression between untreated patients with normal-tension glaucoma and patients with therapeutically reduced intraocular pressures. Am J Ophthalmol 1998; 126: 487–497.

Ensuring accurate Goldmann tonometry

Accurate and methodical technique is the key to good Goldmann tonometry. As with every technique, practice is key.

Technique

The tonometer head should be sterilized in an appropriate solution for an appropriate length of time (check local policy for precise details of sterilization technique). Alternatively there are disposable tonometer heads available.

The patient should be seated at the slit lamp and the procedure explained to the patient.

A drop of topical anesthetic is instilled into the eye. The patient should be warned that the drop will sting slightly but reassured that it will numb the eye fully.

Fluorescein now needs to be applied to the eye. Either a combination fluorescein/topical anesthetic drop should be used or a fluorescein strip may now be applied to the inferior fornix. The patient is encouraged to blink and then any excess tears are mopped up by the examiner.

The dial should be set to 10 mmHg and the biprism/tonometer head should be aligned with the center of the cornea. The cobalt blue filter should be turned up to full illumination and the largest beam possible used.

The patient should be encouraged to fixate a point behind the examiner ensuring that the eyes are kept in the primary position of gaze. The patient should be advised that the eye is now numb but the lids are not. If they maintain their eyes wide open they will not feel anything.

Ease the apparatus slowly forward until the tonometer tip is in contact with the cornea. If the patient cannot maintain their eyes open the examiner should gently help them. It is important to avoid pressure upon the eye as this may result in an artificially increased IOP.

Looking down the barrel of the biprisms you will see two yellow–green fluorescent semicircles. Adjust the slit lamp until the two semicircles are equal in size and well centered. Turn the dial until the inner borders just meet. You will note that the semicircles will oscillate (bounce) back and forth with each ocular pulse. Choose the point where the inner borders meet at the midpoint of this movement. At this point the applanation area is optimal. The force (in grams) being applied by the tonometer head is now exactly (in theory) one-tenth the intraocular pressure (IOP) in mmHg. Now read the dial and multiply by ten to give the IOP.

Several readings should be taken to ensure consistency and accuracy.

Potential errors

If the semicircles are too narrow (i.e. not enough fluorescein on the eye or very poor tear film) the IOP will be underestimated. If the semicircles are too wide (too much fluorescein on ocular surface) then overestimation of IOP can result. In addition vertical misalignment, excessive corneal curvature or abnormal shaped corneas may result in inaccuracies. Previous manipulation of the eye (such as gonioscopy) or repeated measurements may 'massage' the eye and inadvertently lower the IOP.

Calibration

It is vital that the accuracy of the GAT is maintained by regular calibration. It is recommended that this procedure is carried out once a week:

1. Turn the dial to the 4 mmHg position. Place the tonometer on the slit lamp as if you were about to take a measurement.
2. Twist the dial anti-clockwise until the head rocks backwards. Check the dial – it should move at the zero point.
3. Move the dial clockwise again until it rocks forward again. It should again move at the zero point.
4. Attach the calibration rod to the tonometer. Align it with the mark one away from the center mark.
5. Check that the head is leaning backwards.
6. Move the dial clockwise until the arm rocks away from you. It should read just above 20 mmHg and make the transition just as the dial hits the '2' mark.
7. Move the dial back again and the head will rock backwards again. It should move when the dial is just below or at 20 mmHg.
8. Adjust the calibration rod to align the mark farthest from the center of the calibration rod, i.e. move the body of the rod towards you.
9. Check that the head is leaning backwards again.
10. Move the dial clockwise until the head rocks away from you. This should be at 60 mmHg.
11. Slowly rotate the dial counter-clockwise until the head rocks backwards again. It should read just below 60 mmHg.

If it calibrates incorrectly it will need to be returned to the manufacturer for recalibration.

Problems

Inappropriate or repeated measures may result in a corneal abrasion. If this occurs then a short course of antibiotic ointment is indicated.

Pathogens such as hepatitis B, adenoviridae, herpes simplex virus and potentially HIV may be isolated from the ocular surface. This emphasizes the need for strict adherence to hygiene and sterilization protocols.

Prion protein diseases such as Creutzfeldt-Jakob disease have led to concerns regarding the re-use of devices which contact the eye. If a patient is known to have a neurological disease it is prudent to use a disposable prism.

Index

Please note that references to non-textual information such as Figures or Tables will be in *italic* print.